Pra
COMPASSIC
IN TIBETA

T0160505

"Yonten, the founder of the Tibetan Healing and Wellness Center in Bangalore, India, and his amanuensis, Weaner,translate and comment on the ancient treatise called the rGyud-bZhi to explain to doctors the Buddhist intellectual foundations of Tibetan medicine.... Yonten's enthusiasm for emotionally committing to patients is compelling, and practitioners may find it inspiring.... A passionate case for alternative medicine with a deep spiritual cast."
— *Kirkus Reviews*

"*Compassion as Remedy in Tibetan Medicine* is a beautiful work that stands on its own in the field of medicine and should inspire countless physicians throughout the world to set their practice within the sphere of compassionate heart, combined with intelligence, pure intention, skillfulness, diligence, and social ethics. It might be considered as a Buddhist equivalent to the Hippocratic Oath, albeit much vaster and deeper in its scope, since it describes various kinds of physicians from the superior ones who give us the means to free ourselves from the causes of suffering, to the ordinary ones who focus only on addressing immediate illnesses. In doing so, Dr. Jampa Yonten, who has himself centered his medical practice around compassion, has made a beautiful gift to our modern world, which is much in need of the 'good heart' advocated by His Holiness the Dalai Lama."
— Matthieu Ricard, author of *Altruism, The Power of Compassion to Transform Ourselves and the World*

"This book will benefit all readers, including physicians, healthcare practitioners, patients, and those who are interested in maintaining good health, which is based on the practice of compassion along with neuroscience." — Dr. Tsewang Tamdin, Visiting Physician of His Holiness the Fourteenth Dalai Lama

"In this book, many personal anecdotes bear testimony to the power of healing when the motivation of the doctor is that of genuine compassion towards the sick. I highly recommend this book to doctors of all persuasions, both modern and traditional." — Geshe Dorji Damdul, Director, Tibet House, New Delhi

"In this context, Dr. Jampa Yonten—[drawing from his time] dealing with various types of patients, in a very experiential manner interspersed with many moving anecdotes—has brought out all Compassionate aspects of healing and the healer in this book. A must-read book for all healthcare practitioners worth their compassion." — Dr. Dorjee Rabten Nyeshar, CMO, Men-Tsee-Khang, Bangalore

"In this book, Dr. Yonten highlights unconditional love and unbiased compassion, two of the most important inner ingredients in the Traditional Tibetan Medicine practitioner's toolbox. Therefore, all healthcare professionals must integrate these into their practice to benefit both themselves and their patients." — Sonam Dorjee, Science Pala (Father of Science), first Tibetan physicist in exile

COMPASSION AS REMEDY IN TIBETAN MEDICINE

HEALING THROUGH LIMITLESS COMPASSION

Dr. Jampa Yonten
WITH Kyle Weaner

FOREWORD BY
H.H. THE DALAI LAMA

Monkfish Book Publishing Company
Rhinebeck, New York

Paperback ISBN 978-1-948626-92-7
eBook ISBN 978-1-948626-93-4

Library of Congress Cataloging-in-Publication Data

Names: Yonten, Jampa, author.
Title: Compassion as remedy in Tibetan medicine : healing through limitless
  compassion / Dr. Jampa Yonten with Kyle Weaner ; foreword by H.H. the
  Dalai Lama.
Description: Rhinebeck, New York : Monkfish Book Publishing Company, [2023]
  | Includes bibliographical references.
Identifiers: LCCN 2022048538 (print) | LCCN 2022048539 (ebook) | ISBN
  9781948626927 (paperback) | ISBN 9781948626934 (ebook)
Subjects: LCSH: Medicine, Tibetan. | Medicine, Tibetan--History. |
  Traditional medicine--Tibet Region.
Classification: LCC R603.T5 Y67 2023 (print) | LCC R603.T5 (ebook) | DDC
  610.951/5--dc23/eng/20221205
LC record available at https://lccn.loc.gov/2022048538
LC ebook record available at https://lccn.loc.gov/2022048539

Book and cover design by Colin Rolfe

Monkfish Book Publishing Company
22 East Market Street, Suite 304
Rhinebeck, NY 12572
(845) 876-4861
monkfishpublishing.com

CONTENTS

DEDICATION

This book is dedicated to the most compassionate being,
His Holiness the Fourteenth Dalai Lama.

"I believe that at every level of society—familial,
tribal, national, and international—the key to a
happier and more successful world is the growth of
compassion. We do not need to become religious,
nor do we need to believe in an ideology. All that
is necessary is for each of us to develop our good
human qualities. I try to treat whoever I meet as
an old friend. This gives me a genuine feeling of
happiness. It is the practice of compassion."
—His Holiness the Fourteenth Dalai Lama

FOREWORD

Tibetan medicine is one of the greatest legacies of Tibetan Buddhist civilization. It is a holistic healing system, deeply influenced by Buddhist practices, that stresses the interdependence of mind, body, and vitality. Tibetan medicine is an integrated system of healthcare that has served the Tibetan people, Mongolians, and people of the Himalayan region well for many centuries. I believe it can still provide much benefit to humanity at large.

Over the years, there have been growing interest in and recognition of Tibetan medical tradition (*Sowa-Rigpa*) among many other communities. Therefore, this book, *Compassion as Remedy* by Dr. Jampa Yonten, will be helpful in providing an opportunity for interested readers to appreciate this valuable but sometimes overlooked aspect of Tibetan cultural heritage and what is being done to preserve it and make it more widely available.

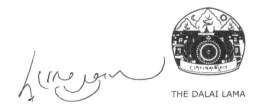

THE DALAI LAMA

—*His Holiness the Fourteenth Dalai Lama*
February 1, 2020

PREFACE

This book is based on the wisdom found in the *rGyud-bZhi* (The Four Tantras), which has been the guiding treatise for Traditional Tibetan Medicine for more than 2,500 years. Of the four sections of the *rGyud-bZhi*—"The Root Tantra," "The Explanatory Tantra,""The Secret Tantra," and "The Last Tantra"—we will focus here on "The Physician Chapter," the final chapter of "The Explanatory Tantra." This chapter teaches the ethics that are essential for physicians and focuses on the development and practice of compassion as well as the pathway to Buddhahood as the great Medicine Buddha. Moral development and the practice of compassion should be of great importance to all medical practitioners and "The Physician Chapter" provides us with detailed instructions.

Three significant stages in my life highlight the profound inspiration that brought me to the study and practice of Tibetan medicine. These stages have inspired me to cultivate the great qualities of a physician in my practice of medicine. The vast meaning and vital importance of "The Physician Chapter" underlies all of these.

When I was in high school in Mussorie, a small town located in the state of Uttaranchal in northern India, I wanted to become an engineer, so my main subjects of study were physics, mathematics, and chemistry. One day I saw a clipping from a newspaper posted on our school bulletin board. It showed a picture of a single hand holding the wrist of another hand with a caption stating that a Tibetan physician can know everything through pulse reading. This sparked my curiosity to study Traditional Tibetan Medicine.

My dream of becoming a Tibetan physician took me to Men-Tsee-Khang (Tibetan Medical and Astrological Institute) in Dharamsala, North India, a great distance from my home in Mundgod in South India. I arrived full of excitement and great hopes for beginning my training, only to learn that admissions were already closed and would not open again for another three and a half years.

Stunned and deeply disappointed, I hardly knew which way to turn. The officials at Men-Tsee-Khang asked where I was from. When they realized how far I had traveled to learn, they offered to let me take an entrance examination in order to become an accountant at the institute. Although it seemed like a diversion from my goal of becoming a physician, I accepted their kind offer. Out of many applicants, only a few were chosen, and I had the good fortune of being one of those. So, working by day in the office as an accountant, I began taking private medical classes at night, awaiting the possibility of the next round of admissions. This was how my dream of becoming a physician slowly grew into a reality.

During that time, the former director of Men-Tsee-Khang, T. J. Tsarong, was organizing an international conference on Traditional Tibetan Medicine in New Delhi. As I was keenly interested in medical studies, I volunteered to assist him. As a result, I was able to attend the conference, where many senior physicians spoke on various topics pertaining to Traditional Tibetan Medicine. Dr. Lobsang Tenzin (Gen Rinpoche) gave a talk on the actions and qualities of a physician based on "The Physician Chapter" of the *rGyud-bZhi*. I had always felt that the deeper meaning and calling of a physician was about generating the qualities of great compassion, love, and care toward suffering beings. My experience at the conference strengthened my passion toward this noble profession. This was the first stage in my journey: It felt as if a confirmation of my destiny had been revealed to me, turning my already deep interest into a deeper respect, a reverence for the profession.

The second stage of my experience with the "The Physician Chapter" came after I had begun my formal studies of Tibetan medicine at Chagpori Tibetan Medical Institute in Darjeeling, India. We were researching commentaries written by great scholars of the past in order to enrich our understanding and to clarify the meaning of this text. As I spent many hours first memorizing and then dissecting each sentence to determine the meaning of the often-encrypted verses (known as *shloka*), a deeper meaning of this valuable subject arose within me.

I was also fortunate during that time to have Dr. Trogawa Rinpoche, the founder of Chagpori Tibetan Medical Institute, as my teacher. He was a brilliant and inspiring example of a physician who was constantly giving love, care, and great compassion to all sentient beings. Many patients told me that just being in his presence made them feel better. At that stage I had been given the knowledge and the means to begin practicing as a physician, but it was not until I actually began practicing that I was able to fully embody the truth of this invaluable teaching.

The third and final stage for me has been realizing, through direct experience, the absolute importance of compassion in the practice of Traditional Tibetan Medicine. I started the Tibetan Healing and Wellness Center in 2003 in Bangalore without any publicity or concrete business strategy. My deep faith in the Medicine Buddha, blessings from my teacher, Dr. Trogawa Rinpoche, support from my well-wishers, my own spiritual practice, and, of course, my recollection of everything that I had been taught by my remarkable teachers, enabled me to offer my healing to people around the world. In these competitive and challenging times, while dealing with patients from different nationalities and backgrounds, I have been able to realize the importance of applying what "The Physician Chapter" teaches—particularly the profound importance of loving-kindness and compassion.

According to Traditional Tibetan Medicine, compassion is the most important quality of a physician. During my visit to Croatia in 2000, a journalist asked me what my specialty was. I quickly responded, "Compassion." The more I practice and travel abroad, giving teachings and consultations, the more I realize the importance and benefits of compassion. A medical practitioner must be motivated to care for every patient who approaches them, regardless of the time it takes, responding with a deep sense of compassion to their physical and mental suffering. It is through the practice of compassion, along with unswerving faith and determination, that my medical practice has benefited many patients around the world.

I hope my readers will benefit from these interpretations of this profound treatise and from my experiences in medical practice. This is my humble perspective of the ancient knowledge and should not be taken as the only way of explanation. If there are any mistakes, please accept my apologies and let me know by writing to me at drjyonten08@gmail.com.

—*Dr. Jampa Yonten*
May 2022

ABOUT THIS BOOK

This book is a translation of and commentary on "The Physician Chapter" from the fundamental Tibetan medical text, the *rGyud-bZhi*. It offers readers a flavor of the richness of Traditional Tibetan Medicine, whose uniqueness lies in the combination of medicine and Dharma.

By integrating healthcare practice with spiritual practice, this book provides guidelines for ethics, the development of wisdom, and the essential role of compassion in healing.

Today, medical practitioners and their patients around the world have taken an increased interest in holistic healing traditions. Their motivations are validly based on the pursuit of natural, noninvasive remedies with fewer side effects. This book reveals how compassion itself can be a primary source of the alleviation of suffering.

Dr. Yonten includes current examples from his clinical practice, from cross-cultural perspectives, and from neuroscience, giving readers a rare and broad view of compassion as remedy. In the words of His Holiness the Fourteenth Dalai Lama, "The ideal physician is one who combines sound medical understanding with compassion and wisdom."

INTRODUCTION

His Holiness the Fourteenth Dalai Lama was once asked what surprised him the most about humanity. His response was: "What surprises me most about humanity is Man, because he sacrifices his health in order to make money. Then he sacrifices money to recuperate his health. And then he is so anxious about the future that he doesn't enjoy the present; the result being he doesn't live in the present or the future; he lives as if he's never going to die, and then he dies having never really lived."

In our modern world, most healthcare practitioners focus on treating a patient's illness with diagnoses and procedures and spend less time understanding and working directly with a patient's experience of their illness, but a patient's underlying, innate illness encompasses so much more than external symptoms and includes their feelings and personal circumstances. As a result, patients often feel neglected and misunderstood. Modern healthcare practitioners are not necessarily lacking in compassion, but their training and understanding of illness focuses their attention and priorities elsewhere, and they struggle with the pressures and stressors inherent in current healthcare systems.

We often hear stories about people whose experience at a hospital became transformed due to the kindness of one particular healthcare practitioner—a single individual can truly make an exceptional difference in a patient's experience.

In Traditional Tibetan Medicine, these qualities are taught and practiced as a standard. Recognizing the preciousness of other sentient beings immediately generates compassion and a sense of caring.

Compassion is essential for understanding and healing our own problems as well as those of others. It is a natural, innate, and instinctual aspect of our being and is first generated from our personal experience of suffering, then from witnessing the suffering of others, and eventually, it is amplified by gratitude. It can be easily experienced by thinking of our parents and others who have nurtured us—our teachers, children, and friends. Ultimately, compassion arises spontaneously, without cause or condition, and is the aspect of our hearts and minds that naturally generates warmth and caring for other beings.

One can train in compassion by regarding all sentient beings as precious. His Holiness the Dalai Lama offers this sage advice from his commentary on the *Eight Verses for Training the Mind*:

> Whenever I interact with someone,
> May I view myself as the lowest amongst all,
> And, from the very depths of my heart,
> Respectfully hold others as superior.

The foundation of this kind of caring is not based on pity. Some of us may confuse compassion with pity, where we distance ourselves from those who are suffering and often look down upon them and their condition. This is not compassion. We can cultivate a deep sense of caring about all sentient beings by recognizing their preciousness.

Compassion is a form of caring that can light up our lives and break open our hearts. When we look at a mother bird feeding her young or animals protecting their babies in the wild, we are moved by these examples of great caring. Consider the heartfelt compassion we feel when we see someone experiencing extreme pain. It is this deep caring that binds us to all that lives. This shared love and pain that we feel in our hearts results from this bond we share with all life.

In Traditional Tibetan Medicine, compassion is a prime ingredient. Whether we are dealing with the details of our daily lives or contemplating ultimate liberation from suffering, it is compassion that inspires us to seek harmony, meaning, and peace. In this tradition, we view our own lives to be just as vital, necessary, and worthy of celebration as we do the lives of others. We see the practice of compassion emerging not just as a remedy for physical ailments, but also as a powerful form of love, care, and affection that sustains ourselves as well as our families, our neighbors, and all of society, extending out into the universe and beyond.

This book is a humble attempt to emphasize some of the great wisdom found in the *rGyud-bZhi* (pronounced *Gyushi*), the fundamental Tibetan medical treatise, which has been the basis of Traditional Tibetan Medical practice for more than 2,500 years.

The English translation of the *rGyud-bZhi* is The Four Tantras; the complete title of the book is *Nectar Essence of the Eight-Branch Secret Oral Instruction Tantra*. "The Physician Chapter" in the *rGyud-bZhi*, which is the focus of this book, is taken from the last of eleven sections of learning found in "The Explanatory Tantra," the second of the four tantras. It teaches the ethics and morals that are essential to Tibetan physicians and focuses on the development of compassion and the attainment of Buddhahood as the great Medicine Buddha. This chapter on the development of the physician holds great importance among Tibetan medical practitioners.

It is said that the Medicine Buddha dwells in the hearts of Tibetan physicians as their guide, mentor, refuge, and aspiration.

The practice of the Medicine Buddha, which is integral to these teachings, will guide us towards developing the necessary skills for becoming deeply compassionate medical practitioners. The instructions provide a clear and thorough explanation of the necessary qualities that a practitioner must possess and how to generate these desirable qualities in body, speech, and mind. For all who seek to heal themselves and others, the practice of the Medicine Buddha is regarded as one of the most profound teachings in the *rGyud-bZhi*. The benefits of following this practice are not only intended for physicians and healthcare providers but for all suffering beings. Its wisdom and compassion are boundless.

—*Dr. Jampa Yonten (Menrampa)*
Physician of Tibetan Medicine
Tibetan Healing and Wellness Center
Bangalore, Karnataka State, India

TRADITIONAL TIBETAN MEDICINE

A Brief History of Traditional Tibetan Medicine

According to Traditional Tibetan Medicine:

The first disease is Indigestion.
The first cause of disease is the Earth element.
The first physician was Jivaka.
The first patient was Shepo.
The first medicine offered was Boiled Water.

This list is a reference to the origins of Traditional Tibetan Medicine and the basis of the lineages in Tibetan culture that were entrusted to propagate this profound healing tradition across the generations. According to Tibetan medicine, the principle of maintaining a strong digestive metabolism remains the basis for physical strength and immunity from disease.

The history of medicine in Tibet predates the establishment of Buddhism in the region. At that time, the Bon religion and culture were dominant in Tibet. As was true with many early indigenous healing systems around the world, the early Tibetan people practiced medicine using herbal, mineral, and animal products. They also used therapies such as minor surgeries and cauterization to bring healing.

The Buddhist system of healing entered Tibet from India in the fourth century. The first physician of the Tibetan lineage was Dung Gi Thorchog. This lineage was then passed down through the royal physicians over many generations. In the eighth century, King Trisong Deutsen organized the first known international medical conference, where physicians from India, China, Persia, and Greece gathered to explore differences and similarities in their healing methods. Later, Yuthog Yonten Gonpo the Elder, also known as the Father of Tibetan Medicine, compiled and wrote the *rGyud-bZhi*, the fundamental Tibetan medical text, along with many medical commentaries on topics such as integrated medicine, pulse reading, and urine analysis. During this time, physicians were trained either through the lineage system or educated in the monasteries.

In the twelfth century, Yuthog Yonten Gonpo the Younger, thirteenth in the lineage of Yuthog, was regarded as another great physician. He traveled throughout the neighboring countries studying medicine and participating in medical conferences with physicians of other traditions. He discovered important connections between the various traditions, thus turning the Tibetan medical system into an integrated system. As a result of the findings he compiled during his lifetime, he rewrote what is the present-day version of the *rGyud-bZhi*.

During the sixteenth and seventeenth centuries, many great scholars from this lineage contributed to the growing wealth of texts and commentaries on medicine and healing. In 1696, Desi Sangye Gyatso, under the auspices of the Fifth Dalai Lama, established Chagpori Drophenling Datsang in Lhasa, Tibet. It was the first official school for Traditional Tibetan Medicine and was intended for the training of monks. During his tenure as the head of Chagpori, Desi

Sangye Gyatso wrote many commentaries on Tibetan medicine and astrology. He also commissioned renowned *thangka* painters to create illustrations of the complete Tibetan healing system, and so established very poignant visual images that physicians and medical students still refer to today.

In 1916, under the great vision of the Thirteenth Dalai Lama, the Tibetan Medical and Astrological Institute, Men-Tsee-Khang, was established in Lhasa. It was the first official medical school for lay people and served as a public health initiative.

In 1959, when China invaded Tibet, the Chagpori Medical School was completely destroyed and many of the physicians were imprisoned, tortured, and killed. Texts and thangkas, which held profound insights into medicinal plants and healing concepts, were also lost in the devastation. After the Chinese occupation of Tibet, His Holiness the Fourteenth Dalai Lama fled to India along with many Tibetans. In 1961, His Holiness established Men-Tsee-Khang in exile at Dharamsala, India, with a few students and teachers. Dr. Trogawa Rinpoche, one of the few Chagpori lineage physicians who escaped to India, was one of the first teachers to teach and practice at the newly established Men Tsee Khang. In 1992, in order to preserve the Chagpori lineage, Dr. Trogawa Rinpoche took great initiatives to establish the Chagpori Tibetan Medical Institute in Darjeeling, India, where I had the great honor to later study and practice.

In India, there are currently four major schools that provide training in Traditional Tibetan Medicine: Men-Tsee-Khang (Tibetan Medical and Astrological Institute) in Dharamsala, Chagpori Tibetan Medical Institute in Darjeeling, the Central University for Tibetan Studies in Varanasi, and the Central Institute of Buddhist Studies in Ladakh. Each of these institutions offers education based on the standards

of the Central Council of Tibetan Medicine, an organiza-
tion that was established in 2004 by the Central Tibetan
Administration. Today, Traditional Tibetan Medicine continues to grow and expand due to globalization with many
new schools arising in and beyond Asia.

A Brief Introduction to Traditional Tibetan Medicine

Traditional Tibetan Medicine is called *Sowa Rigpa*, which
means "the science of healing." Sowa Rigpa is an integrative,
holistic, and profound system consisting of eight branches
of medicine, eleven sections of learning, fifteen occasions
of healing, and four sutras of explanation. Sowa Rigpa can
be distilled into understanding the basis of a healthy and
unhealthy body, the actions and methods of healing, and the
qualities of a physician. This book explores the six categories of the actions of a physician: the qualities, nature, definition, classification, functions, and results of the physician. In
order to provide some background for this important topic,
what follows is a brief introduction to Traditional Tibetan
Medicine.

In Tibetan medicine, the origin of disease is understood to
be ignorance (*marigpa* in Tibetan), which means to not know
the true nature of the self, or else engaging in self-grasping. Ignorance presents itself as 84,000 mental afflictions.
These can be condensed into 404 disorders, and then further
divided into four types of illnesses: karmic, spirit-related,
miscellaneous, and humor disorders. These 404 disorders all
manifest in the body and mind based on the three humors:
rLung (pronounced *loong*), or wind; *mKhris-pa* (pronounced
tripa), or bile; and *Badkan* (pronounced *bay-ken*), or phlegm.

The cause of disease is the most important thing for a
Tibetan physician to understand because without uprooting

the cause one can never be truly free of suffering. The ultimate cause of disease, as stated above, is ignorance. This is generally manifested as the three unhealthy states of the mind, which are called the three mental poisons: desire, aversion, and delusion.

Tibetan medicine further lists four conditional causes of illness, which are season, spirit, diet, and lifestyle. These conditional causes, along with the mental poisons, bring about diseases or disturbances in the balance of the three humors, *rLung, mKhris-pa,* and *Badkan* (wind, bile, and phlegm respectively), which arise in the body and mind. These diseases are diagnosed by the three systems of seeing, touching, and interrogation, and are then followed by the four types of treatments of diet, lifestyle, medication, and therapy, accompanied by spiritual practices.

> *True health is a state of physical, mental,*
> *and spiritual well-being, and not merely*
> *an absence of pain.*

The Uniqueness of Traditional Tibetan Medicine

Ultimately, the key to Traditional Tibetan Medicine, and what sets it apart from other medical systems, whether allopathic, homeopathic, Traditional Chinese Medicine, or Ayurvedic, is the practice of Buddhadharma, or Buddhist philosophy. This practice is based on the understanding of the relationship between the body, the mind, and spiritual practice.

The Tibetan medical system developed alongside Buddhism in Tibet, and as a result, the Tibetan physician placed great emphasis on the practice of the Medicine Buddha. This deeply experienced knowledge of the power of the Medicine Buddha is very significant in the practice of

Tibetan medicine. The power of the Medicine Buddha motivates all aspects of healing: the medical student's training, the physician's treatment, the effectiveness of treatment, and the patient's understanding and ability to benefit from the treatment.

Once this is acknowledged and understood, it's easy to see why Tibetans, especially medical practitioners, believe that Sowa Rigpa is one of the most profound healing systems. Sowa Rigpa utilizes the wise and compassionate healing of the Medicine Buddha (*Sangye Menla* in Tibetan), which means awakened healing.

The integration of this spiritual aspect of healing affects the physician's motivation, conduct, and goals in daily life. The physician who authentically participates in this practice with sincere devotion comes to embody limitless and total compassion towards all sentient beings. As the physician develops within themselves the qualities of the Medicine Buddha, every thought, word, and action—every moment—becomes an opportunity for awakening and benefiting sentient beings. The Medicine Buddha and his emanations of blue healing light becomes a source of healing in the physician, who in turn offers boundless energy to benefit others.

A Prayer to the Medicine Buddha

Compassionate Buddha
Who benefits sentient beings by your virtue,
Hearing your name will prevent suffering.
Medicine Buddha, who dispels
The illness of three mental poisons,
I prostrate to you, the king of Lapis Lazuli light.

"If you want others to be happy, practice compassion.
If you want to be happy, practice compassion."
—His Holiness the Fourteenth Dalai Lama

THE PHYSICIAN CHAPTER OF THE *RGYUD-BZHI*

In the *rGyud-bZhi*, "The Physician Chapter," which covers the prerequisite qualities that are essential for an eminent physician, is part of the final section of "The Explanatory Tantra." This chapter is also known as "Actions of a Physician."

This important chapter is taught by two sages who engage in a dialogue that reveals the wisdom of the Tibetan medical system. In "The Root Tantra," these two sages emanate from the Medicine Buddha according to what the Buddha wishes to teach. It is said that the first sage, Rig-pai-Yeshes (Wisdom Light), emanates from the Buddha's heart, though later, in "The Explanatory Tantra," it is mentioned that he emanates from the Buddha's crown chakra. This sage teaches us the knowledge of the science of healing.

The second sage, Yid-les-sKyes (Born of the Mind), appears to emanate from the Medicine Buddha's tongue, and is the sage who questions the first sage and requests that this knowledge be revealed. These two sages are both the essence of wisdom. One has the wisdom to ask the correct questions, and the other has the wisdom to fully answer these questions.

The teachings are given in the form of verses and bear profound meaning. Throughout the book, I have delineated the different sections of "The Physician Chapter" by highlighting these root verses (in *italics*), and then explaining them so that the depth of this wisdom may be more easily understood.

Dialogue Between the Sages

The second sage, Yid-les-sKyes, asks the first sage, Rig-pai-Yeshes, to reveal the knowledge of the science of healing:

> *"Oh, respected revealer sage, Rig-pai-Yeshes, how*
> *should one learn the actions of the Physician? Great*
> *healer Medicine King, please explain."*
> *When asked, the revealer replied:*
> *"Oh great sage Yid-les-sKyes, what you asked is,*
> *'Who is the healer whose actions heal?' The section*
> *on 'Actions of a Physician' will be shown."*

Yid-les-sKyes respectfully asks, "How should one learn the actions of the physician?" Here the sage is inquiring about the professional, ethical, and personal characteristics, as well as the tasks involved in the practice of healing. The emphasis is on the importance of the interaction of the physician with the patient, where the physician possesses the knowledge and practical aspects of medical treatment.

Rig-pai-Yeshes responds with respect, addressing Yid-les-sKyes as a great sage. He then begins to clarify the question by replying, "What you asked is, who is the actual healer whose actions heal?" This looks directly into identifying who is trained as a healer, who acts as a real healer, and who is successful in healing. This question opens the way to determining the inner experience of the healer, the healer's actions, and the healer's behavior as qualifiers for being a great healer.

The sage Rig-pai-Yeshes then continues: "In the section on 'Actions of a Physician,' the wholesome Physician is revealed under six categories: the qualities, the nature, the definition, the classification, the functions, and the results."

Here the sage lays out the six categories of the actions of a wholesome physician that are to be followed. From this point onward, it becomes the singular voice of the sage, Rig-pai-Yeshes, revealing the instructions and meaning of the actions of the physician.

The sage Yid-les-sKyes is simply listening and asks no further questions. What follows is the main instructions and meaning of the entire chapter, with each category shown separately to make understanding more accessible.

"Only the development of compassion and
understanding of others can bring us
the tranquility and happiness
we all seek."
—His Holiness the Fourteenth Dalai Lama

Chapter 1

THE QUALITIES OF A PHYSICIAN

"The six prerequisite qualities of an eminent Physician are: being intelligent, having a compassionate heart, having pure intention, being skillful in all works, being diligent, and being an expert in social ethics."

Six qualities are required for a person to qualify as a physician, regardless of how much knowledge, technological expertise, or professional experience they possess. Since these qualities are vital to both the experience and the transmission of deep healing, they are referred to as the prerequisite qualities. The six prerequisite qualities are: intelligence, a compassionate heart, pure intention, skillfulness, diligence, and social ethics.

INTELLIGENCE

"From those qualities, the first is intelligence. Within that there are three types of intelligence: broad-mindedness, stable-mindedness, and deep-mindedness."

The first quality, intelligence, seems quite natural. One must have a high degree of intelligence in order to complete the arduous hours of study and acquisition of knowledge necessary to practice medicine. The text illuminates three aspects of intelligence: broad-mindedness, stable-mindedness, and deep-mindedness.

Broad-Mindedness

"One thoroughly understands every detail of the
healing science and medical treatises,
leaving nothing out."

This aspect of intelligence encompasses not only the memorization of medical texts, but also a complete integration of the material so that it becomes familiar, clear, and easily accessible. The physician should possess the capacity to recall medical knowledge swiftly and fully when a situation presents itself. To engage even more fully in broad-mindedness, the physician must be able to adapt the medical knowledge when conditions are not presented exactly as they are in the text. The physician must also be able to apply the teachings to any type of situation that might arise.

For example, many patients come to my office complaining of either hypothyroidism or hyperthyroidism. This is a diagnosis that has been given by an allopathic physician, describing the physical condition of the patient based on medical history, physical examination, and laboratory tests. The Tibetan system of the *rGyud-bZhi* does not describe a specific gland that determines the energy level and metabolic state of a person. What it does describe is the metabolic condition as observed by pulse, urine, and physical characteristics. It is necessary to see if the problem is hot or cold.

In general, hypothyroidism is connected to a cold condition, and hyperthyroidism to a hot condition. Since this relates to the weight of the individual and to metabolic function, it is considered within the realm of *Badkan* and *mKhris-pa*, so we treat hot and cold conditions accordingly. Through a thorough understanding of the teachings, the physician is able to adapt to modern times and contemporary illnesses. It's important to integrate science with the changing conditions of our patients as well as with the world we live in, while still relying on the wisdom training of our text and tradition to support, guide, and direct our efforts.

Tibetan physicians in today's world familiarize themselves with Western medical reports so that the information given by the patient can be understood and utilized. Similarly, allopathic physicians might choose to become familiar with traditional, alternative, and complementary systems so that they too can understand other treatments that a patient may be undergoing. This benefits both the patient and the physician. In this manner, the physician first learns their own system thoroughly, and then becomes familiar with other systems in order to exhibit broad-mindedness.

Stable-Mindedness

"One gives practical treatments without any
feeling of apprehension."

Stable-mindedness encompasses a wide range of mental and emotional attributes, including a strong sense of confidence, emotional stability, and clarity of mind. In a state of stable-mindedness, it's possible to give practical treatments without difficulty or feelings of inferiority. When a treatment involves surgery or the elimination of pus, the physician does not become repulsed or upset. The stability of the physician inspires the patient's confidence in the treatment. In cases where a course of treatment demands an immediate decision, the physician's stable mind can easily and smoothly respond with complete competency. When the treatment involves focused attention over an extended period of time, the physician is not distracted or tired. These are small examples of how possessing stable-mindedness helps a physician.

Stable-mindedness depends largely on the ability to maintain single-pointed concentration. This can and should be cultivated. Our modern times are filled with many distractions, so I highly recommend the cultivation of these grounded mental states, which can easily be achieved with a regular meditation practice.

In recent years, meditation and mindfulness practices have become popular in Western culture. This is, in part, due to the numerous research studies that have shown the practical benefits of these practices as well as the science behind these benefits—the actual changes that occur in the brain. One study, for example, compared performances on a cognitive test given in the face of many distractions. It was found that seasoned meditators, compared with those who never meditated before, made fewer errors.[1] Subsequently, when some of the nonmeditators were taught to meditate in an eight-week program, their performance improved, showing that with training, this skill can be learned.

My colleague Dr. Julie Brefczynski-Lewis, a neuroscientist, assisted with brain imaging studies at Dr. Richie Davidson's laboratory at the University of Wisconsin, where

---

[1] Jha, A.P., Krompinger, J. and Baime, M.J., 2007. Mindfulness training modifies subsystems of attention. *Cognitive, Affective, & Behavioral Neuroscience* 7(2), pp.109-119.

they studied meditation practitioners with 10,000 to 50,000 hours of meditation practice. Their findings offer insight into the state of stable-mindedness. In one study, they found that the level of brain response to a simulated depiction of suffering depended on the type of meditation practice the participants were doing. When seasoned meditators heard a woman screaming in distress while engaging in compassion meditation, they had a stronger emotional response in the brain compared with nonmeditators.[2] However, when they switched from compassion meditation to concentration meditation, their emotional reactions to the distressing distraction decreased considerably and, in some cases, there was no emotional response.[3]

The concentration meditation study was criticized by some people who thought this restrictive response to suffering indicated that it lessened their empathy for suffering. But these critics didn't know about the findings from the study in which these same meditators, upon hearing the same distressing sounds while engaging in compassion meditation, showed even more activation in emotion and empathy-related brain regions than nonmeditators did. Dr. Brefczynski-Lewis suggests that one of the skills that results from these meditation practices is a capability to have both a nimble and stable mind, where it's possible to change emotional responses as needed, and not become uncontrollably carried away by an emotional response. This kind of grounded and flexible mental stability

[2] Lutz, A., Brefczynski-Lewis, J., Johnstone, T. and Davidson, R.J., 2008. Regulation of the neural circuitry of emotion by compassion meditation: effects of meditative expertise. PloS one, 3(3), p.e1897.
[3] Brefczynski-Lewis, J.A., Lutz, A., Schaefer, H.S., Levinson, D.B. and Davidson, R.J., 2007. Neural correlates of attentional expertise in long-term meditation practitioners. Proceedings of the National Academy of Sciences, 104(27), pp.11483-11488.

would be very useful for a physician who wants to empathize deeply with their patients, but also needs to have a clear and stable mind to make quick and accurate decisions without becoming distracted by their emotions and the environment. This would also be an important skill for preventing burnout, as it would offer some protection against becoming debilitated and numb from overexposure to suffering.

I will now briefly describe a concentration meditation practice that is easy to do. To develop single-pointed concentration, simply focus on any one of the five senses. Let's take the sensation of feeling as an example. Concentrate on the feeling of the breath in both exhalation and inhalation. At this time, do not try to control the rhythm or strength of the breath, just feel the breath fill and empty itself. When there is no longer any internal or external disturbance that can distract from the observation of this feeling, this is the attainment of single-pointed concentration.

When beginning this practice, it is very common to encounter numerous distractions of thoughts or emotions. This is because the mind is habitually not calm. Maintaining a calm state is extremely important for stable-mindedness.

Let us again take the breath as an object of meditation. In this case, naturally inhale and then exhale a relaxed breath. Before the next inhalation, just observe the sensation of being completely empty of breath. Notice if there is any thought or emotion when the breath is fully exhaled. Then, without forcing, take a natural inhalation. Do this several times, pausing after a relaxed exhale. Observe the experience after exhalation, and then naturally inhale. Notice if the mind is becoming more relaxed, quiet, and peaceful.

These methods of meditation will help in the development of a stable mind. It can be done every morning or evening or whenever it's convenient. However, meditation is never practiced in the presence of the patient—when with the patient, a physician's focus should always be completely on the patient and the task at hand. The research has shown that the effects of meditation done regularly will carry over to activities performed during the day. Finally, do not become distracted with the thought that you must meditate in order to have a stable mind. Simply do the practice.

Furthermore, the physician should rely upon the foundation of knowledge that is developed in the first category of broad-mindedness. Faith in the true, clear knowledge of the medical text naturally leads to stability and confidence. This stability is accomplished through the practice of the six perfections: generosity, morality, tolerance, diligence, meditative concentration, and wisdom.

In this way, the physician maintains a firm concentration, along with devotion to the lineage and service to all suffering beings.

Deep-Mindedness

"One uses analytic wisdom, which helps to
develop clairvoyant wisdom for offering
a clear diagnosis and prognosis."

The third quality, deep-mindedness, utilizes analytic wisdom in order to attain a state of clairvoyance. By clairvoyance, we are not referring to a mystical, magical practice, but rather to the ability to see ahead and know clearly. The deep-minded physician cultivates mindfulness while remembering their teacher's instructions, and thus attains great confidence in practice. Therefore, in Tibetan Buddhism, according to the *rGyud-bZhi*, the elements of deep-mindedness are categorized as the lineage, the wisdom deities, and the protectors.

The wisdom deities are aspects of our own minds. They are symbolic of the dynamic aspects of compassion and awareness, and are inseparable from our innate potential, our teachers, and our lineage. While the visual images of the wisdom deities such as the Medicine Buddha are often associated with religion and culture, they are in truth much more profound than this. Our minds naturally work with images and symbols, such as in dreams, memories, and thoughts. The deities are particularly significant symbols that help us to overcome our self-centeredness, emotional fixations, and frozen perceptions of ourselves, our lives, and how the universe is. The wisdom deities invite us to connect with the basic goodness, intelligence, and openness that naturally exist within us and in all sentient beings.

The protectors are often depicted as frightening characters dressed in flames or animal skins, bearing fierce expressions and postures. These images are also beyond culture, religion, and ethnicity. They are archetypal forms that represent the more subtle energies of human existence. Their purpose is to communicate and connect directly with these energies, particularly our negative emotions, in order to uproot and transform them.

The protectors evoke and encourage discipline and devotion within the practitioner, and help pacify physical, emotional, and environmental obstacles. They help to restore vision and equanimity, so that we can see all situations as workable. They are dynamic and help us to realize our own flexibility and strength, building confidence and determination.

The physician's reliance on spiritual practice, teachers, and deities generates deep-mindedness. This leads to the attainment of clairvoyance, which is important to the ability to identify the root cause of a disease and make a prognosis for its treatment.

According to Buddhist tradition, clairvoyance (*Ngon-Shes* in Tibetan) is attained as the result of highly developed meditative concentration. It is often considered to be the awakening of the third eye, or the divine eye. The tradition is very clear about the power of clairvoyance and it is categorized into six types: divine eye, the ability to observe the suffering of others; divine ear, the ability to hear even the minutest sound of insects and understand the different languages of all living beings; the knowledge of gauging others' thoughts and emotions; knowledge of miracles, the ability to perform supernatural deeds; the knowledge of the past and future; and lastly, knowledge of the decay and destruction of the negative passions in order to purify the body and mind. These six types of clairvoyance can only be understood by someone who has achieved a high level of meditative concentration. They are stated here in order to show the extent of the capabilities that can manifest in the physician with this attainment.

Let us come to a practical understanding of the idea that analytical wisdom can bring us to a state of clarity. We will use medical practice as an example. As the physician becomes more sensitive to subtle signs, more and more subtle levels of awareness are attained. Eventually the physician is able to make a diagnosis, determine the treatment, and make a prognosis of the outcome with great detail and accuracy.

The power of clairvoyance is connected with the law of interdependence. It is possible to see how the impact of clairvoyance reaches down to the cellular level and relates to receiving messages in the body from the greater world. The exterior body and environment acts as a mirror of the internal state.

It has only been in the past fifty years or so that medical practitioners have relied on technology for diagnosis. Before this, physicians used their own skills of observation, experience, and deduction to make a diagnosis. Ideally, these skills are applied along with the use of modern technology to support diagnosis and treatment.

For the development of clear seeing, begin with gross observations and slowly move towards more and more subtle ones. Look at the appearance of the skin, sense organs, and excretions, and how they present. Then pay close attention to the voice, breath, movement, and finally the mind.

The external environment can also present reflections in the same way, offering the physician a wealth of knowledge related to diagnosis and treatment. In Traditional Tibetan Medicine, we can see signs in the surrounding environment or phenomena that occur, which help us to determine how successful the treatment will be. This is a display of how the internal and external are so closely related and interdependent.

The idea of clairvoyance may seem questionable to some readers. It's unfortunate that we have mostly dismissed the idea that human consciousness can operate in these subtle ways, despite the fact that many of us have coarser experiences of this in our daily lives. Intuition, for example, is a common experience. We often have clairvoyant experiences, premonitions, or dreams about people we know, or about situations and events, which are, in fact, signs about what is happening, or about to happen. Through meditation and the development of awareness and concentration, we can become more sensitive to subtle communication, signs, and conditions.

Someone who truly has clairvoyance has attained it through diligent practice and the development of wisdom. This wisdom can also be used to determine the correct times to reveal these realizations. This ability is called skillful means. A deep-minded physician thoroughly understands all the phenomena and can use wisdom to discriminate in determining the right time to reveal insights and interpretations to the patient.

"Out of all the prerequisite qualities,
intelligence is considered the best."

A skillful physician cultivates these three aspects of intelligence: broad-mindedness, stable-mindedness, and deep-mindedness. Intelligence is the most important of all the prerequisite qualities because it leads to the wisdom of unwavering analytic understanding. These qualities provide the foundation for a student to complete their study of medicine, and for a physician to continue with both their practice and teaching of medicine. The accomplished physician will be able to practice by truly understanding the nature of the disease and by using all medical procedures known, to arrest the disease without any doubt. This clear knowledge, based on analytic wisdom, brings forth courage, enthusiasm, and confidence in the practice. The qualities involved in the deeper aspects of intelligence will completely sustain the physician throughout a life of practice.

COMPASSIONATE HEART

"A compassionate heart means to have
bodhichitta (Buddha mind). There are three
practices for developing a compassionate heart:
the preliminary practice, the main practice,
and the dedication practice."

The first practice, the preliminary practice, emphasizes the generation of a wish to help eliminate suffering and to maintain pure faith in the Three Jewels of Buddhadharma. The second, the main practice, consists of the practice of the four limitless qualities. The third practice of dedication requires the physician to engage in continuous practice, while embodying the virtues of the medical tradition and upholding equanimity towards all beings in all circumstances.

A compassionate heart is saturated with the mind of bodhichitta, which fully embodies kindheartedness. The term in Tibetan is *Sampa Karwa* (*bsam pa dkar ba*) and it translates as "white mind." As will be explained, this compassionate heart of bodhichitta, the wish to benefit others, emerges from a twofold recognition: first, to recognize the suffering of others, and second, to realize the interrelatedness of self with others.

Buddhism posits that when the physician sees others in pain, they can actually feel what their patients feel.

Notice that we are saying, "We *feel* the suffering of others," and not "We *think about* the suffering of others." What happens when we experience feelings? Are there physiological reactions? When we love someone, how do we experience that love? Do we experience love in the heart? We use the phrase "kindheartedness" for a particular reason. "Kindness" means having a kind and sympathetic nature, and "heart" indicates the place where kindness comes from. It is not simply a thought or idea, but rather there is an actual and palpable feeling in the experience.

Neuroscience research has confirmed that viewing others who are suffering or feeling happiness activates the brain in the same way as if we were actually experiencing the pain or joy.[4] The degree of similarity between viewed pain and actual

---

[4] Singer, T. and Klimecki, O.M., 2014. Empathy and compassion. *Current Biology*, 24(18), pp.R875-R878.

pain depends on a physician's capacity for empathy. In the West, this empathic experience of pain can lead to feelings of distress. But many experienced meditators have developed the skill of stable-mindedness, and as a result, not only are they not disabled by these feelings of empathic pain, but they are also inspired and capable of responding to whatever is needed to help others.

This idea brings us back to the core of Tibetan medicine, which is the body and mind connection associated with kindheartedness.

In medicine, we work to end the suffering of others through the administration of medical procedures, and through a kind heart, which extends warm and pleasant feelings to our patients. We hold the well-being of others as more important than our own, since we know that our well-being is dependent upon their well-being.

Imagine a world where no relief from suffering can be found. Everywhere people's expressions reveal deep sorrow, unhappiness, frustration, and anger. We would most likely be fully drawn into this world of negativities. Now imagine a world filled with compassion and benevolence, where everyone is smiling and emanating loving-kindness like His Holiness the Dalai Lama constantly does. This would be a world filled with great happiness and joy.

A compassionate heart holds the key to understanding how we live and work, and how our brains and our physiology impact both ourselves and others in all aspects of our lives. The compassionate heart is an expression of our brains and emotions working at their very best. We want to see others in a state of well-being, since their health and happiness creates the same feeling in us. This is the core of Tibetan medicine, the body-mind connection, and it is expressed as the compassionate heart of bodhichitta.

After we fully recognize and open ourselves to the suffering of others, then follows the realization of our interrelatedness with all others. We are intricately connected with every other person we see, not only through shared feelings, but also through the very essence of our beings. Our identities are not as separate from those around us as we may think.

Consider how much the attitude of your physician affects your experience. If your physician seems genuinely happy, compassionate, and caring, it is more likely that you will enjoy the visit and feel better. The physician's capacity to connect with the suffering of patients and to be able to experience this suffering as their own, aids in the patients' recovery. This empathy, appearing on the face of the physician, immediately brings about a sense of relief to the patient and increases feelings of well-being. The compassionate heart is a powerful method for relieving the pain and suffering of patients.

As we all go through the stages of birth, illness, old age, and death, and embrace a deeper understanding of our connection with all life, we come to see that the nature of suffering is the same for us all. From this understanding we develop a kind and compassionate heart.

These contemplations inspire us to work to benefit others in a balanced state of equanimity, without any bias or differentiation between patients, without praising some and blaming others.

Having discussed the compassionate heart from the view of the two aspects of recognizing the suffering of others and understanding interrelatedness, we now turn to the three practices: the preliminary practice, the main practice, and the dedication practice.

The Preliminary Practice

"First is the preliminary practice of observing suffering, developing a wish to help others, maintaining faith, and keeping equanimity between good and bad, love and hate."

The preliminary practice consists of four aspects. The first requires us to observe the suffering of all sentient beings. The second requires us to develop a desire to help all of them. The third involves faith, and in particular, faith in the Three Jewels. The fourth involves avoiding discrimination or differentiation between love and hate, war and peace, black and white—essentially, practicing moderation.

A brief survey of the magnitude of suffering may help us to understand more clearly this first aspect of the preliminary practice of a compassionate heart: to observe the suffering of all sentient beings and contemplate the amount of death and sickness that is taking place right now. In every direction, consider how much death is taking place. Think of the bugs and bacteria around you, the birds above, and the fish in the oceans. Think also about the trees decaying and dying or being destroyed. Imagine how many animals are dying across the planet at this very moment. Now include all humans.

None of this is meant to make you feel sad but is rather a clear statement of the truth: that which is born is subject to sickness, aging, and death. The more clearly we see this and recognize the suffering caused by this, the more our hearts grow soft with tenderness for all of life that surrounds us. As we realize that all indeed is passing away, we begin to behold the precious fragility of all life. Since all are subject to this same law of impermanence, all suffer. This knowledge raises our awareness of interdependence, and of how we are all in the same situation, without exception. In this way, we all suffer.

True realization of this shared quality of suffering brings with it the next question: "What can I do to help?" Here begins the second aspect of the preliminary practice of a compassionate heart. From the observance and acceptance of suffering, arises the natural, spontaneous opening of the human heart with a desire to help. This compassion, the openheartedness of the physician, determines the amount of motivation they will bring to their practice of medicine. If seeing suffering evokes a strong feeling to help, then the more suffering that is seen, the more the wish to help will arise. On the contrary, when a physician feels exhausted in the face of personal problems, which comes from viewing the self as independent and separate, the physician will most likely become unable to offer good help and will experience burnout. But with compassion as their motivation, a physician gains great inspiration to help others in their encounters with suffering.

Compassion is considered a limitless quality because it grows the more we practice it. This quality of compassion is essential to a physician of Tibetan Medicine. If a physician possesses all the factual knowledge and medical techniques required for practice, but is lacking in kindheartedness, the traditional teacher will recommend that the student continue in study.

Compassion is the desire to help. The physician is constantly aiming or striving to develop a deeper awareness of the suffering of all beings. Out of this vast ocean of empathy arises the next aspect of the preliminary practice: "What can I do to help ease this immense suffering?"

What a great opportunity! What an exquisite experience! The fragile nature of this fleeting life inspires us to help in whatever way we can. By pushing the boundaries of our sympathy for the fragility of all lives, the first preliminary practice produces a natural empathic response. It is based on the recognition that we are not separate from those "others out there" who suffer. Their suffering is our suffering. By deeply opening our hearts and making room for the intensity of empathy to arise, physicians can truly aspire to help reduce the suffering of others and perfect the art of healing.

The third aspect of the preliminary practice of a compassionate heart is the practice of taking refuge. As we contemplate the constant and unwavering presence of suffering and loss in the world, we may find we need to develop faith. Faith can be generated through the practice of taking refuge in the Buddha, the Dharma, and the Sangha, which means to experience the benefits of the teachings of the Buddha. Without the strength and stability that comes from these teachings which help us to move beyond our limited sense of self, the experience of seeing the suffering of others may be too difficult or overwhelming. Healthcare practitioners lacking this sense of refuge may well experience burnout. As a result in the third aspect of the preliminary practice we are encouraged to become grounded in faith.

Buddhists, therefore, take refuge in the Three Jewels—the Buddha, the Dharma, and the Sangha—so that our own personal desires and self-grasping will not overwhelm the goal of developing the wisdom and compassion for cherishing others. Here I will provide three different interpretations of the Three Jewels in order to give the reader a broader understanding of the practice of taking refuge.

The first perspective comes from a teaching His Holiness the Fourteenth Dalai Lama gave in India in 1960, soon after he came into exile:

"Whether or not you are a Buddhist is determined by whether or not you have taken refuge in the Three Jewels—Buddha, Dharma and Sangha—purely, from the depths of your heart. Simply reciting Buddhist prayers, playing with a rosary or walking around temples does not make you a Buddhist. Even a monkey can be taught to do these things. Dharma is a matter of mind and spirit, not external activities. Therefore, to be a Buddhist, you must understand exactly what the Three Jewels of refuge are and how they relate to your spiritual life.

"With respect to refuge in Buddha, we talk about the causal Buddha refuge—all the buddhas of the past, present, and future, of whom the most relevant to us is Buddha Shakyamuni—and the resultant Buddha refuge—refuge in our own potential for enlightenment, the Buddha that each of us will become. As for taking refuge in Dharma, there is the Dharma that is taught in the scriptures and that which is the spiritual realization of what was taught. Finally, we take refuge in Sangha, in both ordinary monks and nuns, who are symbols of the Sangha, and the Arya Sangha—those beings who have gained direct meditational experience of the ultimate mode of truth. Therefore, we say that Buddha is the teacher, Dharma is the way, and Sangha are the helpful spiritual companions.

"Of these three, the most important to us as individuals is the Dharma, for ultimately only we can help ourselves—nobody else can achieve our enlightenment for us or give it to us. Enlightenment comes only to the person who practices Dharma well, to the one who takes the Dharma and applies it to the cultivation of their own mental continuum. Therefore, of the Three Jewels, Dharma is the ultimate refuge. By hearing, contemplating, and meditating on Dharma, our lives can become one with it and enlightenment can become an immediate possibility."

The second interpretation comes from Professor Robert Thurman, a great scholar and practitioner of Tibetan Buddhism, who has outlined a clear expression of the power of taking refuge in the Three Jewels in simple terms. In his book *The Jewel Tree of Tibet*, he writes the following:

"... Buddha means all those who have awakened from the sleep of ignorance and blossomed into their full poten-tial.... Awakened and blossomed, they are teachers of oth-ers.... We take refuge in the Buddha. We mean, we turn to the teaching of the reality of bliss, the teaching of the pos-sibility of happiness, the teaching of the method of achiev-ing happiness in whatever form it comes to us, whether it comes as Christianity, whether it comes as humanism, whether it comes as Hinduism, Sufism or Buddhism."

One of the meanings of Dharma is "to be held." Thurman continues:

"The highest meaning of Dharma is the reality that is our own reality—the reality that holds us in freedom from suffering, that holds us apart from suffering, holds us in a state of bliss. Dharma is our own reality that we seek to understand fully, to open to fully.... Virtues and ethics and practices are also Dharma. Even the qualities we develop, the positive qualities that lead us toward freedom and reality, those are Dharma. Dharma means more like Joseph Campbell's great statement: Follow your bliss! Bliss is your freedom."

Professor Thurman continues with the third Jewel, the Sangha:

> "The third jewel is the Sangha, the community of those who ... are consciously evolving toward being Buddhas, sharing their understanding and bliss with others, as teachers of freedom to other beings, helping them discover these jewels."

The final interpretation of the Three Jewels comes from Traditional Tibetan Medicine. The refuge of the Buddha that is taken in the medical practice is that of the perfect physician. The refuge in the Dharma is in the teachings of medicine and its practice, specifically the wisdom of the *rGyud-bZhi*. The Sangha includes all those who participate in healthcare practice: doctors, nurses, pharmacists, and caregivers. As we meditate and practice taking refuge in the Three Jewels, we strengthen the positive potential within us, and weaken all negative habituated patterns. We practice this daily, or as often as possible. And just as a practiced muscle grows stronger and an unused muscle grows weaker, in this same way we know without any doubt that taking refuge in the truth of the Three Jewels increases our desire to benefit others and consequently increases our own happiness.

The analytical wisdom in first recognizing and accepting the deep sorrows of the world, and then turning towards it, opens our hearts toward everything that lives. As we feel more connected with all lives, and with the suffering inherent in life, we begin to realize that our own suffering is small compared to the suffering in the world. Suffering, then, is no longer personal—it completely transcends personal space and is seen as a naturally occurring aspect of all life. As this truth works its way into our being, we are offered strength through taking refuge in the Buddha, Dharma, and Sangha.

This practice deepens our empathy for suffering and our capacity for selflessness, while offering us a place of refuge and strength. The result is that the practitioner is not left to drift in the sea of sorrow, but rather, finds the strength to hold on with greater commitment. This is why they are called the Three Jewels, because in the sea of suffering, the visualization and thought of the Buddha, Dharma, and Sangha promotes a feeling of well-being and strength to face the challenges of life. This is very important for all beings and especially for those who tirelessly work at alleviating the suffering of others.

By meditating upon the suffering of the world, our desire to help those who suffer and our commitment to taking refuge will grow stronger. Studies have shown that these skills grow and increase over time by strengthening the pathways in our brain. Small structural changes resulting from repeated meditation sessions, along with the effects of taking refuge, increase the pathways of empathy and interrelatedness. More practice results in larger pathways for experiencing positive thoughts, as well as an increasing sense of strength that is so useful for dealing with the stressors of daily life. This is especially helpful for medical practitioners whose daily lives are surrounded by deep suffering. This inner cultivation of the physician results in the development of a deeply loving, empathic, and caring human being. The compassionate physician knows how to take shelter in the Three Jewels, and how to increase the inner sense of stability and strength. And they truly know that offering themselves to alleviate the suffering of the world is the path toward their own well-being.

The final preliminary practice of a compassionate heart is equanimity. Here, the physician develops a stable mind that avoids differentiation between love and hate, or attachment and aversion. This means, very simply, the physician develops a sense of oneness for all and avoids giving more attention to those who offer praise, money, prestige, or status. The physician will endeavor to be equal in taking care of all beings, regardless of caste, creed, race, gender, religion, or class.

Equanimity extends beyond the relationship of medical professionals with their patients. Equanimity promotes the practice of calm stability in the constantly changing circumstances of life. Whether our experience of the external world is positive, loving, and full of kind people and pleasant events, or is filled with great difficulty, the practice here is to keep ourselves on an even keel. The practice of seeing suffering, developing a desire to help, and maintaining faith in that practice by actually alleviating suffering, evokes a sense of calm balance within the heart and mind. Practicing this over time creates a state of continual balance that will deepen immeasurably.

The Main Practice

"Continually practice the four limitless qualities— compassion, love, joy, and equanimity—as the main practice on a daily basis. This aids in developing the mind of enlightenment."

The main practice of a compassionate heart follows the preliminary practice. The main practice consists of the development of, and continued practice in, the four limitless qualities: compassion, love, joy, and equanimity. As the name limitless qualities implies, these states of consciousness can grow immeasurably.

In preparation for the following exercise, it is important to understand the traditional Tibetan devotion to the mother. Whether the mother referred to is our personal mother or an archetypal mother embodied in a deity such as Tara, Tibetans revere the mother. There is the notion that through the process of rebirth, all beings have once been our mothers during our countless cyclic births. Therefore, all life and all sentient beings deserve to be treated as we would treat our beloved mother.

Whether or not our own mother was overworked, inadequately prepared for parenthood, ambiguous about her role, or perhaps overwhelmed by being the primary caregiver, we can still appreciate the fact that without our mothers we would never have been born. We all can appreciate the love and care that was given to us by a devoted human being, who changed our diapers, fed us, dressed us, and protected us when we were young children.

Recall someone who helped you, who provided you with deep care and loving warmth when it was needed. If this is difficult, begin by contemplating the many qualities of mothering that surround us: nest-building, den preparation, gestation, giving birth, and providing milk. Mothers are the nourishers of a brand-new life, they provide for all forms of life. Then recall how all of us, as sentient beings, are dependent on countless other lives for our survival, nourishment, and happiness. This dependence is like a child's dependence on their mother.

Here, let us concentrate on the four limitless qualities, which are the main practices for developing a compassionate heart. This concise visualization practice is presented for the medical practitioner.

How to Develop the Four Limitless Qualities

It is very important to have an object for visualization: here, let us imagine a sick person who is in great pain. In witnessing this person's suffering, you experience limitless compassion arising and moving throughout your body. This compassion fills you completely and then begins to spill out of every pore of your body into the world and the universe.

Now remember the endless number of beings who have supported and sustained you through your journey thus far and begin to think of them all as your actual mother. Next, regard this sick person as one who has supported you unconditionally, just as a devoted mother would. Now, generate limitless love towards this sick person, by wishing them the happiness that they have been deprived of.

We experience feelings of limitless joy when we engage in the act of freeing a sick person from illness and returning them to happiness. This practice, then, brings great benefits both to ourselves and to others. It is a practice of limitless joy!

Lastly, in doing this, we must take care not to be partial to race, age, gender, wealth, or any other discrimination. Seeing all beings as equally deserving of happiness, our wish is to benefit them all equally. This is the quality of limitless equanimity in practice.

The aspiration of such a compassionate heart will generate the mind of enlightenment, or bodhichitta, through the natural arising of both wisdom and compassion. By deeply looking at the nature of suffering, and realizing the interconnectedness of self and others, we generate wisdom. This wisdom is knowing the impermanence of life, the unity of self and others, and the empty nature of reality. Truly seeing suffering as a natural and constantly fluctuating process helps us to realize impermanence, while seeing the connection between self and others helps us experience interdependence. Ultimately, we become free from the delusion of being an independent, separate entity, and we begin to see the empty nature of reality.

Compassion, the other aspect of the mind of enlightenment, is practiced by wishing to help alleviate the suffering of all sentient beings, and then taking action to do so. This is how we accumulate merit and ripen our minds for awakening. So these two aspects of wisdom and compassion are intrinsic parts of the compassionate heart and are both required to awaken the mind of enlightenment.

When I gave a talk entitled "Compassion as Remedy" at the Lutheran Medical Center in New York City, one resident physician commented that this was all good in theory, but when it came to medicine in the real world, there was never enough time to practice compassion with the high volume of sick and agitated patients. I explained to him that you don't have to stop seeing patients or go somewhere to meditate to feel compassion. In fact, there is no special meditation practice to be done while you are seeing the patient. The physician should, rather, be completely present with the patient in order to figure out how best to improve their state of health and wellness by practicing love, compassion, joy, and equanimity. This is how we can express compassion—by seeing suffering and working to relieve it through love. However, meditating on the generation of compassion on your own, such as the beginning or end of your day, helps you feel more genuine compassion when with actual patients.

The Practice of Compassion

Closing our eyes and taking long deep breaths isn't enough. Compassion is also a limitless quality that will continue to develop the more we engage with it. This is why we set our intention of benefiting others each day before we start work, taking inspiration from the Prayer for the Four Limitless Qualities.

Prayer for the Four Measureless Qualities

May all sentient beings have happiness and the causes of happiness.
May all sentient beings be free from suffering and the causes of suffering.
May all sentient beings never be separated from the happiness that is without suffering.
May all sentient beings abide in equanimity, free from both attachment and aversion.

This is how we set our intention each day. If we have more time, then it is possible to do a longer meditation to deepen the experience. Having explored these limitless qualities in some depth, we can now begin to understand the wisdom of Tibetan medical training and in particular, the main practice of the four limitless qualities.

Dedication

"Continually practice while realizing the virtuous qualities of the medical tradition and treat others without favor or holding any grudge."

This final aspect of the second prerequisite quality, a compassionate heart, teaches us about dedication. Here, the physician trains in returning to the four limitless qualities repeatedly, while remembering the virtuous qualities and actions involved in all the health sciences and medical professions.

Dedication is a gratitude practice guiding the physician to make a conscious recollection of the positive power of this chosen profession.

The physician engages in the practice of equanimity regardless of whether there is praise or blame for their work. In this way, the physician develops an outlook in which they can remain free from holding grudges or indulging in pride when any praise or blame comes from their patients.

If the physician you consult makes you feel that your problems, however small, matter as much to them as they do to you, how can this not affect the outcome? You feel better for being in the presence of someone who deeply and empathically listens and cares for you. You feel better being in the presence of someone you feel deeply connected to. Better yet, if you sense this physician is balanced and possesses some wisdom about life, your trust and respect naturally increases. When we see a physician with a genuinely friendly attitude, someone who welcomes and treats all others with the same caring, we see this person as being mature and completely trustworthy. We find it easy to open ourselves to them fully.

These qualities of a physician deeply impact treatment and often result in a speedy recovery. Therefore, the development of these qualities is paramount in our training as physicians.

Likewise, when physicians practice these attitudes in all aspects of their own lives—when they commit to genuinely practicing compassion, loving-kindness, sympathetic joy, and equanimity—it is guaranteed that they will bring to their work the attitudes and empathy that increase the efficacy of their medical practices.

"Having these aspects of the compassionate
heart ensures easy cures and assists in
the recoveries of many."

This section clearly shows us that embodying these aspects of a compassionate heart, which focuses on the attainment of spiritual qualities, helps in an easier recovery for many patients. Seeing the impact of developing trust and intimacy with patients in my own practice has helped me to recognize the incredible truth of the guidance found in "The Physician Chapter." I know with certainty that practicing compassion works. With no intention of boasting, I can give innumerable accounts of healing difficult and even terminal disorders by simply following these instructions of the compassionate heart. Of course, no one can guarantee a cure for every disease. We have to practice compassion and put all of our effort towards helping others without any expectation of the results. Having a compassionate heart and practicing with it, not only cures diseases, but also makes the patient's visit to the physician a joy.

His Holiness the Dalai Lama often highlights the differences between a physician who may not be an expert but who is capable, kind, and benefits many patients, and a physician who is intelligent and skillful but arrogant. Patients prefer kind physicians because they feel calmer and intuitively experience the compassionate field which expedites healing.

PURE INTENTION

"To have a pure intention, one takes six vows, two commitments, and upholds three wisdoms."

We are about to enter the heart of Tibetan medical training in our exploration of the third prerequisite quality. We take the six vows in order to view the teacher as the Buddha, the teachings as the words of the Buddha, the medical texts as the holy scripts of the Buddha, and our friends in the profession of healing as our beloved Dharma friends or well-loved relatives. We also vow to view all patients as our own children and to regard their pus and blood as if these were fluids from our pet.

The text describes two commitments. The first is to regard the medical lineage holders, the Arya Sangha, as protector deities. The second is that we view all medical instruments as being exactly the same as those of the protector deities— forever ready to protect all suffering beings, anytime and anywhere. These commitments enhance our preparedness, altruism, devotion, and courage while diminishing selfishness, fearfulness, and confusion.

Then we follow the three wisdoms that uphold the sanctity of medicine. The three wisdoms are: to regard the medicines as wish-fulfilling gems that are able to fulfill our patients' wishes for good health; to regard the medicines as nectars that are empowered with the potential to immediately relieve the patients' suffering and prolong their lifespans; and finally, to regard the medicines as the precious offerings we make to the Medicine Buddha and the great sages who have perfected these sciences of healing.

Next, we engage in the practice of visualizing the Medicine Buddha. What is the method of visualization? And how can it help us practice medicine? Human beings are creative and have powerful imaginations. So, our minds naturally work with images, symbols, and sounds. These aspects of the mind exist in all human beings. Visualization can utilize these natural tendencies for positive transformation. With our minds, we envision an image of the Medicine Buddha along with images that are symbolic of primordial healing that benefit all sentient beings. This is clearly not intended for self-empowerment or for self-improvement. We are evoking our minds to manifest the qualities of openness, loving-kindness, awareness, and clarity for the benefit of all suffering beings.

Scientific research has shown that visualization can have an effect on the brain that is similar to actually seeing the object or performing the tasks visualized. Take, for example, a study that asked participants to imagine performing a particular finger movement sequence.[5] In this study, the more vivid the visualization of the finger performance, the more the participant improved in the actual task performance of the finger sequence. In terms of brain activation, if their visualization evoked brain activity that was similar to the activity the real finger performance evoked, their skill improved. Research has also been done with athletes, musicians, and even surgeons to improve their performance through visualizing the skills they wish to acquire in an ideal and successful way.[6]

In Traditional Tibetan Medicine these methods of visualization have been relied upon for centuries and have provided a pathway for the development and realization of countless sages and physicians. What could be more profound than the visualization of oneself as the ultimate of healers, the Medicine Buddha, along with his supreme instruments of healing? This visualization practice of the Medicine Buddha can transform the physician into a Supreme Healer.

Pathways of Transformation

Pure intention (*Dam-Tshig* in Tibetan) plays a very important role in both Buddhism and in Tibetan medicine. It is the

[5] Lebon, F., Horn, U., Domin, M. and Lotze, M., 2018. Motor imagery training: Kinesthetic imagery strategy and inferior parietal f MRI activation. Human brain mapping, 39(4), pp.1805-1813.

[6] Anton, N.E., Bean, E.A., Hammonds, S.C. and Stefanidis, D., 2017. Application of mental skills training in surgery: a review of its effectiveness and proposed next steps. *Journal of Laparoendoscopic & Advanced Surgical Techniques*, 27(5), pp.459-469.

quality that transforms a relationship from being mundane into becoming profound and sacred. Dam-Tshig is often translated as a commitment, devotion, or vow, but here I have chosen to translate it as pure intention. Dam-Tshig involves faith, devotion, loyalty, and trust, all of which lead to a purity in relationship. In Western Medicine, physicians take the Hippocratic Oath which is a commitment to practice medicine with the full intention to help patients and do no harm. The concept of Dam-Tshig is similar but goes deeper, involving the daily practice of cultivating compassion by the physician—they do this practice for themselves, for their patients, and for all sentient beings. The Hippocratic Oath is indeed wonderful and noble, but unfortunately traditionally it's recited only during graduation from medical school and is not reviewed or practiced regularly.

Dam-Tshig develops in the heart. The actions and behaviors that result from it are not felt as obligations or duties. In its presence, spontaneous willingness springs forth without any doubt, grudge, or resentment. Dam-Tshig has a deep meaning that plays an especially important role in the relationship between the teacher and the student. This relationship demands reciprocity: if the student has Dam-Tshig, but the teacher does not, or vice versa, then the relationship and the teaching will not reach its highest potential. It is the same between the physician and the patient.

The full experience of Dam-Tshig blossoms in many aspects of life, not just in the relationship of teacher and student or physician and patient. With Dam-Tshig active in the heart, a person finds the motivation to do whatever is necessary, under any circumstances. We will explore the six vows, two commitments, and three wisdoms that comprise the prerequisite quality of pure intention for a physician so that our understanding of Dam-Tshig deepens.

The Six Vows

"First, one regards the teacher as the Buddha, the
teaching as the Buddha's teachings, the medical text
as the holy scripts of the Buddha, the friends as
Dharma friends or relatives, the patients as one's
children, and the bodily fluids of the patient being
like those of a pet. These six vows should be kept in
mind while practicing pure intention."

The six vows teach us that the Buddha is a model of wisdom and compassion for us to follow. The teachings are seen as the Buddha's teachings in order to increase our sense of faith in the healing abilities we are learning or practicing, and the medical texts are seen as the holy scripts of the Buddha to be treated with respect, dignity, and a sense of the sacredness for all the knowledge imparted. Our fellow students and colleagues are viewed as Dharma friends or relatives who encourage us to interact with loyalty, integrity, and respect. The patient is seen as our own child, which allows for the expression of loving-care, and the patient's bodily fluids are seen as those of a pet, so there is no fear or disgust when we encounter bleeding or infected wounds.

When considering the vow to treat all our patients as if they are our own children, we need to consider modern and cultural differences.

The aim of the training in our traditional system of Tibetan medicine is the development of a wholesome psyche that is based upon compassion, loving-kindness, joy, and equanimity in all life circumstances and extends towards all beings.

In 1989, Dr. Trogawa Rinpoche gave a talk in Baltimore, Maryland. An audience member asked about the potential difficulties of treating patients who are close friends and family, with whom it might be difficult to be objective and maintain a scientific perspective. Rinpoche laughed and said, "Oh yes, in Tibet we have a saying for this: 'Your eyelashes are too close for you to see.'" Rinpoche, however, did treat all his family and himself without this attachment and confusion interfering.

What Rinpoche meant was that the attachment and delusion that the physician has for their relatives and close friends can be so strong that they are unable to see clearly. This is why, in Tibetan medicine, we work on the realization that all beings are interrelated and that all have been our mothers. When we come to this understanding, there will be no sense of attachment or aversion, and all can be cared for equally. Every patient can be considered as dear to us as our own child, but without any emotional attachment that clouds clarity.

From this perspective, it makes sense that the training encourages the physician to see patients as if they are their own children. The same efforts you would make to spare your child of any pain or discomfort and to ensure that they feel loved and comforted: this is what you bring to your patients. Even the very bodily fluids of the patient are to be treated with the same equanimity, not with disgust. This is the essence of mind-training to practice pure intention.

The Two Commitments

"Secondly, regard all medical knowledge holders as protector deities, and their medical instruments as the deities' instruments, ready to protect all suffering beings, anytime and anywhere."

When we view eminent medical knowledge holders as protector deities, they become our fearless protector deities. This enables the physician to confidently make crucial decisions. In the Tibetan medical lineage of spiritual practices, there are nine protector deities called the Dhamchen Degu. These deities are portrayed with bulging eyes and fierce expressions, holding various weapons, sometimes wearing garlands of human skulls around their necks, bodies dripping with blood, and often riding on dangerous animals. On a general level, these characteristics symbolize the deep courage with which they protect all suffering beings and the lineage of medicine. On more specific levels, each aspect of the protector deity represents the practice of that particular deity; for example, Lopon Shanglon is one of the nine deities that removes obstacles.

When we regard our medical instruments as the deities' instruments, we are ready to protect all suffering beings, anytime and anywhere. This is another way of acting with courage, timeliness, and precision. The instruments carried by the wrathful protectors represent different methods of the practice. The *vajra* cutter blade and skull bowl that Lopon Shanglon holds in front of his heart represents the practice of cutting through ignorance with the knife to awaken the inherent wisdom in the skull. Robert Beer explains in his book, *The Handbook of Tibetan Buddhist Symbols*: "When the deity holds the knife above the skull-cup in front of his heart, it symbolizes that method (knife) arises from, and is permeated (blood) with wisdom (skull-cup). It may also symbolize the deity's commitment to his tantric vows (Dam-Tshig), whereby he liberates or revives vow-breakers by metaphorically drinking their blood." Just like the weapons of this wrathful protector are meant for method and wisdom, as well as the upholding of commitments, the physician's medical instruments are wielded with technical expertise and with the pure motivation to help others.

The courage and readiness to practice medicine at any moment stretches us beyond our ideas of having office hours, of being on duty or off duty. Instead, we see our life as being inseparable from being a physician. This gives us courage and an infinite wealth of energy to continue practicing through hardships.

The Three Wisdoms

"Thirdly, regard the medicines as a wish-fulfilling gem, a nectar, and an offering. Medicines are regarded as a wish-fulfilling gem, which will manifest all wishes and desires. Regard the medicines as nectar, capable of instantly curing all the diseases. And the medicines are to be regarded as spiritual offerings offered to the holders of medical knowledge and sages."

We might wonder how our thoughts or meditation on medicine could change its effectiveness. One possible explanation is put forth in the book *The Hidden Messages in Water*, in which author Masaru Emoto and his assistants experimented with how words and emotions might have an impact on water's crystalline structure. When they encouraged water with phrases such as, "Let's do it!" or "Thank you," the crystals became clear, beautiful, and precise. When they ordered the water around or said, "You fool," the crystals were either unformed or deformed. They discovered that water that had been prayed over formed the strongest, most beautiful crystals of all.

Emoto's experiments suggest that water—a common element in the world, including Tibetan medicine—responds with great sensitivity to its environment. Although his study would still benefit from more replication, there is well-vetted science in the field of quantum physics that shows that the observer affects the measurement of how particles of matter behave, and how they affect other particles.[7] In light of this, viewing medicine as a wish-fulfilling gem, as nectar, and as a worthy offering to the holders of medical knowledge makes perfect sense. Believing this, and treating medicine in this manner, enhances its efficacy.

Up until this time, these spiritual practices have been kept secret because of how easily they could be misunderstood and misused. These practices are not based on belief or fantasy, but rather, involve ritual transformations using the mind's intention for the benefit of others. They are meant to, and in fact do, increase the efficacy of the medicine, transforming them from simple compounds into nectar-like gem offerings.

The Method of Transforming Medicines

"First, the precious jewel and medicinal ingredients are sought out and retained. Second, the medicines are well compounded and blessed."

Traditionally, physicians searched in the highlands of the Himalayan regions, particularly the mountains of Tibet, looking for medicinal plants and minerals, especially on auspicious days such as the full moon or new moon, or on the eighth day of the lunar month, which is considered to be Medicine Buddha Day. Their knowledge of botany, geology, and the taste of the medicine and its potencies was highly

---

[7] Weizmann Institute Of Science. "Quantum Theory Demonstrated: Observation Affects Reality." *ScienceDaily*, February 27, 1998.

developed. They understood how the location of each plant and its exposure to the climate changed its potency in important ways. The seeking and retaining of necessary medicinal ingredients is a vast field of knowledge, much more extensive and comprehensive than this brief explanation.

Next, the gathered ingredients are compounded. The process of compounding involves much more than simply combining the ingredients. For many compounds, there are ingredients that need to be extracted, purified, condensed, and calcified. Then the ingredients are weighed and combined according to prescribed specifications. The time of the collection of the herbs and the time of compounding has to be noted, and astrological almanacs must be consulted. The season, moon phase, and stars all play a role in heightening the efficacy of the herb being collected or the compound being made.

Finally, the text states that the compounds must be blessed. This can be done through the visualization practices, invocations, mantras, and healing rituals. It is also done by inviting Lamas and other spiritual practitioners to consecrate them.

"In order to transform medicines, visualize oneself
as the Medicine Buddha, the King of Lapis Lazuli
Light; the medicine as nectar, and the medicine
vessel as the Buddha's begging bowl filled with
nectar. Then recall and invoke the teachers of
medicine and the great sages during the process of
making supplication for this blessing."

This is the process for transforming the medicine from an ordinary substance into a wish-fulfilling gem and a nectar that can give vitality and relieve suffering. It starts with physicians visualizing themselves as the Medicine Buddha.

The vessel that is being used to compound the medicine is visualized as being the same as the nectar-filled bowl that is held by the Medicine Buddha. The lineage of great sages that have mastered the practice of medicine for generations are recalled, as the following supplication is recited and the medicine is transformed and blessed for consumption.

Supplication to the Medicine Buddha

"Healing Buddha, king of Physicians, Victorious
one, conqueror of the three mental poisons,
Teacher—Medicine Buddha, whose incarnated body
has the great names and apparent structure of the
Buddha, and shines a deep blue color, Lapis Lazuli.
In the right hand is held the antidote to suffering
from wind, bile, and phlegm diseases, A-ru-ra,
chebulic myrobalan—the king of medicines. Resting
in the lap, the left hand is holding a begging bowl full
of nectar. I prostrate to the Lapis Lazuli light
of Medicine Buddha."

There are a few preliminary things the practitioner should follow when meditating and visualizing. They should find a quiet and calm place to sit. In order to set the mood and clear out negative energies, light some incense. Take a seat on a cushion which is neither too high nor too soft and then, sit with a straight spine and legs crossed. If sitting in a chair, keep the feet flat on the ground. Then allow the mind to rest in a calm state. Don't follow thoughts of the past or future. Simply come to a quiet place of rest.

Now come the guided instructions for meditation on the Medicine Buddha. This visualization is from a teaching that my teacher, Dr. Trogawa Rinpoche, gave in New York City in 1989.

Visualize the empty space in front of you where the divine form of the Guru Medicine Buddha is seated on a lotus and moon cushion. His body is in the nature of deep blue light, the color of Lapis Lazuli. He is very serene and adorned with silk robes and glorious ornaments made of jewels.

Guru Medicine Buddha's right hand rests on his right knee, palm outstretched in the gesture of giving realizations, holding the Arura, the king of medicines. His left hand rests on his lap in the gesture of meditative equipoise, holding a nectar bowl of medicinal fruits that cures all disorders.

This is followed by a prayer: "May your vow to benefit all sentient beings now ripen for me and others."

Granting your request, from the heart and holy body of the king of Medicine, infinite rays of light pour down completely, filling your body from head to toe. They purify all your diseases and afflictions due to spirits and their attributes, and all your negative karma and mental obscurations. In the nature of his light, your body becomes crystal clear and pure.

The light rays then pour down twice more, each time filling your body with blissful, clean, clear light which you absorb.

At the heart of Medicine Buddha appears a moon disc. Standing at the center of the moon disc, is the blue seed-syllable *HUNG* surrounded by the syllables of the mantra. As you recite the mantra, *Tadyatha Om Beshajay, Beshajay Maha Beshajay, Beshajay Raja, Samudgate*

Svaha, visualize rays of light radiating out in all directions from the syllables at his heart. The light rays pervade all sentient beings of the six realms. Through your great love wishing them to have happiness, and through your great compassion wishing them to be free from all sufferings, they are purified of all diseases, afflictions due to spirits and their attributes, and negative karma and mental afflictions.

Feel great joy and think that all sentient beings are transformed into the Guru Medicine Buddha. How wonderful that I am now able to lead all sentient beings into the Medicine Buddha's enlightenment!

With this merit, may I complete the benevolent actions of the children of the Buddhas, the Victorious Ones. May I become the holy savior, refuge, and helper for the sentient beings who have repeatedly been kind to me in their past lives.

By the virtues of attempting this practice, may all living beings who see, hear, touch, or remember me—even those who say my name—at that moment be released from their miseries and experience happiness forever.

As all sentient beings, infinite as space, are encompassed by the Guru Medicine Buddha's compassion, may I also become the guide of sentient beings existing throughout all ten directions of the universe.

Because of these virtues, may I quickly become Guru Medicine Buddha and lead every sentient being into his enlightened realm.

The physician, by performing this ritual in the early morning hours, is refreshed and becomes more compassionate toward patients. The physician supplicating to the Medicine Buddha is the ultimate practitioner of the profession.

This is the ultimate spiritual practice of a Tibetan medical practitioner. It is essential to accomplish spiritual attainment as the Medicine Buddha, to have complete confidence in oneself as the Medicine Buddha, in order to benefit all suffering beings, especially one's patients.

Supplication to the Great Sages

> *"Sustaining the highest wisdom in all the supreme*
> *eighteen fields of knowledge, receiving mastery*
> *over life through the meritorious result of essence-*
> *extraction, with clairvoyant mind and compassion,*
> *bringing harmony to Supreme Beings: I prostrate to*
> *the sacred wisdom holder sages."*

Another source of inspiration, confidence and strength are the sages of this great lineage, who have developed the highest wisdom in all the supreme eighteen fields of knowledge. This invocation prayer or supplication of respect and reverence is made to the great sages who helped to develop, promote, and protect this great medical lineage. Sages such as Jivaka, Nagarjuna, Yuthog Yonten Gonpo, and Desi Sangye Gyatso are among the many who have contributed to this lineage and stand as profound examples of the mastery of the wisdom of healing. These particular sages provided paths to enlightenment through complete mastery of the body and mind.

> *"Just as the god's nectar, the naga's supreme jewel*
> *crown, and the sage's elixir, you will hold this*
> *medicine close with confidence in its benefits."*

These healing wisdoms transform the consecrated medicine into a nectar that can prolong life and even make us immortal, like the ambrosia of the gods. This nectar is something that can cure any ailment immediately, which is why it is said that the medicine is transformed into the nectar of the gods.

In Asian cultures, the *naga*, or serpent spirit, is associated with protecting great wealth, and is often depicted as having a great jewel in the crown. It has the power to fulfill wishes, and so, when we compare the consecrated medicine to the naga's crown jewel, it is to show the wish-fulfilling capacity of the medicines.

Lastly, the sage who has accomplished all eighteen great sciences, the three types of compassion, the eight accomplishments, and the six clairvoyant wisdoms has the power of the elixir—which is a life-prolonging power. In this way, the medicine that is consecrated by the Guru Medicine Buddha and Lineage-Holding Sages has the ability to prolong life. With all of these qualities, the physician understands that medicine is invaluable and can heal any disease and problem. The medicine is kept physically close to ensure its availability when needed, but more importantly, a deep confidence and faith in its powers is kept close to the heart.

"The four hundred and four diseases of wind, bile,
and phlegm, which disturb the continuity of life, are
pacified. The one thousand eighty mental afflictions,
and the three hundred sixty spirit disorders, which
disturb the mind, are all healed."

This statement shows that the transforming power of these medicines not only helps with physical illness, but also helps with mental illness, emotional disturbances, and harmful obstacles, which can be the primary cause of illness. These divisions are deeply explained in Buddhist scriptures on psychology, as well as in the Traditional Tibetan Medical texts.

The four hundred and four diseases are listed as: one hundred and one diseases due to karma, one hundred and one diseases due to spirits, one hundred and one diseases due to miscellaneous problems, and one hundred and one diseases due to a disturbance of the three humors.

According to Traditional Tibetan Medicine, diseases are not just physical and mental illnesses, but can also be karmic, or due to spirits.

After going to a specialist, many patients come to me and say that they are not improving from their illness. Being a Tibetan physician, I look at the larger perspective of the illness, and sometimes consider the possibility of diseases related to karma. Along with a treatment, we might also suggest spiritual practices, such as chanting healing mantras, prostrations, circumambulations, offerings, and rituals, all of which can help purify karma and thus can aid in a speedy recovery. Spiritual practices like prostrations and circumambulations will benefit karmic disorders of the body, while chanting and prayer will benefit karmic disorders of the speech. Likewise, meditation and visualization will benefit karmic disorders of the mind.

One of my Tibetan patients was suffering from tuberculosis. He was taking Western medicines along with Tibetan medicines to help his immune system and to hasten recovery. He asked me if I thought it might also be a karmic disease. I thought it might be so and recommended practicing prostrations. He started doing prostrations every morning and evening. This helped him tremendously, and he recovered in a short time.

The *rGyud-bZhi* describes five types of disorders caused by *gDon* (elemental spirits). These are: psychosis, amnesia, epilepsy, strokes, and skin and lymphatic disorders such as leprosy. Now, not all of these problems are considered spirit disorders, but we need to be aware that these can be affected by spirit influences. There are many different kinds of spirit-related disorders that must be understood thoroughly in order to help patients suffering from these problems.

One of my teacher's patients was diagnosed with a life-threatening disease—lymphocytic lymphoma of the non-specific nodular type. What follows is based on an account from the first *Chagpori* newsletter.

Ernest Scharag, a research scientist, was put on drugs that made him sick during his stay at Boulder Memorial Hospital. As a result, he was desperately looking for alternative therapies. It was around that time that my teacher, Dr. Trogawa Rinpoche, was visiting the hospital to offer consultation and seminars on Traditional Tibetan Medicine. In the course of his consultation with Ernest, Rinpoche asked him if he had ever lived in the mountains or moved any white stones. Ernest replied that he had moved from the city to New Mexico, where he had picked up some white quartz stones to decorate his ranch. Rinpoche told him his condition was related to removing the stones which had stirred up a snake spirit, a naga, that dwelled there.

Ernest was prescribed the following regimen: He was to perform specific spiritual practices on a daily basis, and perform an annual ceremony to the snake god, Naga, once a year. He was to take three types of herbal medicines three times a day, consume the precious jewel pill every month on the new and full moon, and follow a prescribed diet. Ernest's health steadily improved. Today Ernest leads a healthy and normal life that includes fundraising for Chagpori Tibetan Medical Institute as an act of gratitude.

Miscellaneous diseases are normally not very serious and can be cured through diet, lifestyle, and positive thinking. Let's take a headache as an example. It might be worth taking a moment to analyze the cause of the problem before simply popping a pill. The cause of the headache may be due to stress, overeating of oily foods, or not sleeping enough. If the headache is caused by stress, then positive thinking and relaxation may relieve it. Drinking lots of boiled warm water for overconsumption of oily foods will help ease the digestive system and eventually the headache. The headache might also be cured by taking a nap and resting, which can help to overcome a headache caused by sleeplessness. It is very important that we don't get anxious and consume pain medicines the moment we feel sick. Instead, we should take some time to look at ourselves to see if our problems might be caused by a faulty diet and lifestyle.

The 101 diseases based on the three humors are categorized in the following ways: forty-two *rLung* (wind) disorders, twenty-six *mKhrispa* (bile) disorders, and thirty-three *Badkan* (phlegm) disorders. These disorders can be addressed and pacified with the four branches of treatment: diet, lifestyle, herbal medications, and therapies.

The 1,080 mental afflictions and the 360 spirits of disturbing emotions, all of which obstruct the mind, can be pacified through the Medicine Buddha practice.

The Sacred Healing Mantra

Om Namo Bhagavate, Beshajay
Guru Baidurya, Prabha Raja, Tathagata
Arahat Samyak Sam Buddha
Tadyatha, Om Beshajay, Beshajay
Maha Beshajay, Beshajay Raja
Samudgate Svaha

This is called the "sacred healing mantra" because it is the essence of the Medicine Buddha practice. If, due to a busy schedule, it becomes difficult to find enough time to recite the longer version of the healing mantra, then by all means, it's possible to recite the short healing mantra, which also has great benefits. Reciting either the long or the short mantra daily—three times, seven times, 108 times, or as much as possible—is beneficial.

Short Healing Mantra

Tadyatha Om Beshajay, Beshajay
Maha Beshajay, Beshajay Raja
Samudgate Svaha

Translation of the Healing Mantra

Om—A pure and auspicious word
Namo—To prostrate or bow respectfully with the body, mind, and speech
Bhagavate—Great Lord or Teacher
Beshajay—Healer, Medicine Buddha
Guru—Teacher, Master
Baidurya—Deep blue, the color of the Lapis Lazuli gem
Prabha Raja—King of Light
Tathagata—Thus Gone One (an epithet of the Buddha)
Arahat—Destroyer of mental poisons
Samyak Sam Buddha—Awakened One or Perfectly Enlightened One
Tadyatha—As it is
Om—Pure, Auspicious, Noble
Beshajay, Beshajay—Healer, Medicine Buddha
Maha Beshajay—Great Healer, Great Medicine Buddha
Beshajay Raja—King of Healers, The King of Physicians
Samudgate—The supreme heights
Svaha—An auspicious word that ends the mantra: So be it!

The Meaning of the Healing Mantra

Noble One! I prostrate to you the Great Master, Medicine Buddha, King of Lapis Lazuli Light, Thus Gone One, who conquers mental afflictions and disorders, the awakened and realized Buddha. As it is. Noble One, Medicine Buddha, Great Medicine Buddha, King of Physicians, Perfectly Enlightened One. This mantra ends with auspicious aspiration. So be it!

Benefits of the Healing Mantra

> *"Reciting this seven times, while visualizing*
> *medicine as a nectar offering to the medicine*
> *knowledge holders, results in the meritorious act of*
> *purifying one's own diseases and dispelling spirit*
> *problems. Those patients who are dying can save*
> *their lives by taking this medicine and reciting this*
> *sacred healing mantra. With complete devotion,*
> *one can achieve blessings, prosperity,*
> *and meritorious results."*

The benefits of these practices have been realized by the great masters of the past, and have been explained to us in this text, but knowledge of these practices should not be taken as dogmatic truth. Buddha said that his words should not be followed blindly, but should be analyzed and tested, just as a goldsmith pounds gold to determine its authenticity.

The human psyche is deeply based on symbolism, and these methods of practice are used to cut through the constraints of our ordinary mind in order to come face-to-face with the primordial mind. The Medicine Buddha image has thirty-two major and eighty minor signs, each representing a specific aspect of enlightenment. The blue color of his body represents the vast expanse of the primordial healing wisdom that is attained in the state of enlightenment. The hand gestures symbolize specific qualities of generosity: the right hand is holding the medicinal plant, Arura, the king of medicine; the left hand, in the gesture of meditative equipoise, is holding a nectar bowl: the nectar signifying meditative accomplishment, and the begging bowl, renunciation.

When we fous on the Medicine Buddha, we are aspiring for the perfection of wisdom to manifest as the unsurpassed, accomplished, and compassionate healer. We are seeking support in healing both ourselves and others from Medicine Buddha, whose healing energy pervades all time and space. Ultimately, we must learn to develop and embody these qualities in ourselves through regular and, eventually, continuous practice.

We are aligning ourselves with what we know to be positive, loving, and wise behavior. We are strengthening our capability to respond with calm serenity, no matter the circumstances. By meditating with trust and confidence, we exercise our inherent potential for wisdom, compassion, and caring devotion as depicted by the Medicine Buddha.

During meditation practice, we are awakening our potential for profound healing wisdom in order to help others in times of need. This is not an intellectual experience, but a dynamic one that engages us with direct experience.

When we meditate on the Medicine Buddha, we use our body, speech, and mind to chant the short healing mantra: *Tadyatha Om Beshajay, Beshajay Maha Beshajay, Beshajay Raja Samudgate Svaha.*

This combination of sacred syllables is an invocation of healing. It allows us to elicit clarity and engage in compassionate action. We focus repeatedly upon the figure of the

Medicine Buddha offering the healing Arura plant from his open palm and holding the medicine bowl of nectar. We unite ourselves with the qualities of supreme powerful healing, and the union of compassion, wisdom, and generosity, through the archetype of the Medicine Buddha's utterly balanced figure.

It is quite possible that because of the physician's strong belief in the medicine and conviction in its efficacy, this will be transmitted to their patients who are then healed. Faith and conviction play an important role in the healing process.

It is natural for us to have doubt. We are encouraged to question authority, results, findings, and old beliefs— to question all junctures of our activity. This questioning has provided us with profound discoveries and continues to push science and medicine towards the edge of the unknown. Nevertheless, we may also benefit by a practice that allows us to sit quietly, contemplate serenity, and deepen our calm. This is also a kind of exploration, but one that focuses on direct inner experience, rather than on intellectual examination of the physical world. When we recite the ancient Sanskrit mantra and visualize and feel the healing blue light pouring down from the perfected being into our own bodies, does it help us? Do we feel any sense of peace, healing, or purification?

The meditation on the Medicine Buddha encourages us to feel calm, compassionate, generous, and joyous, enjoying our natural state. We visualize the image of the Medicine Buddha, study his expression, and find his serenity. We can find healing in the pure blue color of Lapis Lazuli. The color blue signifies a vast, deep, and endless knowledge of healing, like the limitless blue sky.

In Tibetan medical practice, the physicians and staff members begin each day with prayers of aspiration for the well-being of others, and with the recitation of healing mantras, prayers, and visualizations of the Medicine Buddha. This is an effective way to set intention at the beginning of the day. I always begin my practice in this way.

So we have developed pure intention through the six vows, the two commitments, the three wisdoms, and through manifesting ourselves as the Medicine Buddha. If we practice these on a daily basis, they will give us infinite strength to continue our practice of medicine tirelessly in order to heal suffering beings.

SKILLFULNESS

"There are three kinds of skillfulness; these are through the body, speech, and mind."

Skillful Body

"One has to be physically skillful at making the medicines and medical instruments as well as at performing the therapies."

The physician has competency in making the medicines and instruments. The traditional way to prepare medicines is to separate the useful parts of the plant, clean them, and then compound them (often using a mortar and pestle or other grinding device). There are many types of instruments used in treatment, such as the cupping bowl, the cauterizing copper, and the golden needle for acupuncture. The physician not only knows how to use them, but knows exactly what they are made of, how they should function, and possibly how to make them.

Once, when we were compounding medicines, our teacher, Dr. Trogawa Rinpoche, came in while sewing some medicine

bags. We were all surprised to see that a Rinpoche was sewing. But Rinpoche told us that a good physician should know
everything, including stitching. If we know how to stitch well,
then in the same way, we should be able to perform surgeries,
along with therapies like enemas, venesection, moxabustion,
and cauterization, with physical grace and accuracy.

In each discipline of healing, be it medicine, nursing, or
physical therapy, there is a body of knowledge, a set of skills,
and a physical manifestation that the practitioner embodies
to transmit to the sick person. The *rGyud-bZhi* advocates
mastery of all these skills for the benefit of others.

Skillful Speech

"The quality of speech is gentle and soft,
which gives joy to the patient."

This skill is very important in relating to patients. The way
we speak, the tone, the word choice, and the body language
all affect the listener greatly. If a physician uses harsh words
or a loud tone, then the patient may leave feeling bad. When
the physician is in a hurry and speaks too quickly or in an
urgent tone, it could aggravate the wind humor in sensitive patients, making them feel agitated instead of calm. So
the physician needs to speak gently, and always be sensitive
to the patient's feelings. This should be true, not only with
patients, but with all those around us. If a physician speaks
softly with patients in the clinic and then uses aggressive and
harsh words outside, it is not only hypocritical and harmful
for their reputation, but it may even inhibit their ability to
practice medicine.

When I was in Dharamsala there was a famous female
Tibetan physician named Ama Lobsang. Everyone loved her

because she was not only an expert physician, but she also spoke gently and softly with great love and care. Everyone talked about her compassion and the gentle way that she spoke, which made patients feel better and happier.

Skillful Mind

> "To have a skillful mind it must be clear, sharp, and without ignorance."

The physician develops these qualities through mind training, by meditation and practice. Possessing a skillful mind is important because that is how we can see clearly what the patient is really experiencing. Sometimes a patient will only share limited information, and at those times, a physician needs to remain very focused and observant in order to sense subtle signs. This can be especially important in cases of previous trauma or abuse, sexual disorders, addictions, and many other situations.

Whatever the physician sees, hears, and thinks is observed and interpreted with clarity. The physician needs the mental sharpness to observe the symptoms, recognize the disease, and determine the treatment, all in a short time, without any doubts.

> "Having all these skills in body, speech, and mind, one becomes the leader of all."

In combination, the body, speech, and mind make up the whole of the individual; thus, being perfected in all these skills will create the best possible physician.

DILIGENCE

"The diligence of a Physician is in two forms:
diligence with respect to oneself and diligence
with respect to patients."

Diligence with Respect to Oneself

"With respect to oneself, one is diligent in the cause
to study, in the condition of having a perfect teacher,
in maintaining the surroundings of good friends,
and, finally, in the diligence of habituation."

The Cause of Study

"The cause of study is to become a qualified
Physician, which is dependent on the perfection
of the grammar in reading, writing,
and understanding of medical texts."

Being a qualified physician means being dedicated to alleviating the suffering of patients, their families, communities, and, in fact, all sentient beings. At its most basic level, all of this is dependent on gaining knowledge of grammar in reading and writing in order to understand medical texts. The physician is then able to decipher the deeper meaning of the poetic verses of the traditional texts.

If we do not have mastery of grammar and spelling, then the meaning can easily be misunderstood. Whatever we do, from the very beginning of study, it is very important to gain and apply clarity of understanding. The ability to explain, argue, and write will make it possible to apply this wisdom.

Becoming accomplished in reading and writing will ultimately determine whether we will gain mastery in medicine or not.

The Condition

"The condition is finding a perfect teacher. There are three aspects of being diligent in the conditions of having the perfect teacher, which are: the qualities of a perfect teacher, the method of following a perfect teacher, and the purpose of having a perfect teacher."

Without the teacher, the student would not be able to learn, and so here, the teacher is considered to be the condition. In Tibetan culture, the students are primarily dependent on the teacher, not only for knowledge, but also for their personal development. So here in Tibetan medical training, the teacher is paramount. Because of this, the student chooses the ideal teacher and seeks to emulate them in the areas of professional practice and character. Thus, the student is entering into an apprenticeship that encompasses medical training as well as character building.

I am fortunate to have had a great teacher, Dr. Trogawa Rinpoche, who was not only a great physician but also a reincarnated Lama who carried the lineage of Chagpori.

When I was working in the Chagpori clinic under Dr. Trogawa Rinpoche, I got to see how Rinpoche was so fearless and gentle in his practice. On one occasion, there was an old woman with cancer who had been visiting our clinic for consultations. We tried so hard to help her with many medications, but with little results. Rinpoche came by, so we requested him to see the patient. He carefully examined her and then prescribed a small dosage of a very common medicine. We were all surprised, but when the patient came back a week later, she had improved considerably. Rinpoche was a very simple, gentle, and compassionate physician and teacher. When we were students, we would sometimes feel that Rinpoche's teachings went too deep, as he would sometimes focus only on one subject and go into great detail about every aspect of it, not seeming to care whether we completed the full curriculum for the course or not, while other teachers would teach very quickly, and cover all the required subjects. Now, as a physician, I can look back at those qualities of his and see how fortunate we were to have such a wise teacher.

The Qualities of a Perfect Teacher

"The perfect teacher possesses the qualities of amassing a vast knowledge of medicine and its practice, is skillful, holds the secret transmissions of the medical practice, is tolerant, is non-materialistic, and is loving, caring, respectable, and worthy of veneration."

The first thing novices look for in a teacher is their clear motivation to teach; we need to know they aren't teaching just for the sake of money, fame, or any other ulterior motive. Whenever we see a wise teacher who possesses pure motivation, we should seek to learn from them. Even a child can become an expert by learning under such a purely motivated and wise teacher.

The teacher should have heard, read, and studied all of the necessary texts and commentaries so that they can explain each word of the text and any part of the medical practice to the student. The teacher should also have received oral instructions and lineage secrets from their teacher on the skills of applied medicine. The teacher should be an expert in diagnosis, therapies, and treatments. The teacher should be tolerant with all beings, especially with patients and students. This is important so that all the actions of healing and teaching can be successful. And finally, the teacher should be non-materialistic. This does not mean that they should be poor or without wealth, but rather, that money and wealth are not their primary goal; also, the teacher should not be miserly or cunning in financial dealings.

Our teacher, Dr. Trogawa Rinpoche, possessed all of these qualities. He was serene and compassionate. He received all the necessary transmissions, initiations, and empowerments, and was highly skilled in medical diagnosis and the compounding of medicines.

Once Rinpoche came to visit our medical school before we left for the final medical examination in Dharamsala. He asked after the well-being of all the students. We told Rinpoche that one of the students had a fever and was sleeping. Rinpoche went to visit him and looked into his eyes and at his tongue to discover that the student had a heart disease. He then asked all of us to check the student's pulse, and to recognize and correlate the pulse reading with the heart disease.

The student was later taken to the hospital and diagnosed with a heart problem. This came as a great awakening to us, to witness Rinpoche's skill in diagnosis.

The Method of Following a Perfect Teacher

"The method of following a teacher is to entrust oneself to the perfect teacher without any doubts.

All work is accomplished without being deceitful.
All behavior is to be modeled after the teacher, and
adjusted according to the teacher's wishes. One feels
an enduring gratitude all the time."

Being able to fully trust the teacher comes from first seeking a perfect teacher, by recognizing their worthiness. Once that is done, there should be no doubt in what the teacher advises. Even if it seems like the teacher is saying something bad or wrong, one can take each word and learn from it.

I was not the best traditional medical student, but I tried to follow my teacher's words very seriously. I traveled abroad, with permission from my teacher, and started my center in Bangalore with his blessings. I always thought of my school and the lineage, and I felt deep gratitude for having the opportunity to study medicine. Today, I feel proud when I go back to my old schools, and they are happy to see me carrying on the lineage. This is a very important aspect of *Dam-Tshig*— the pure relationship between teacher and disciple that is filled with trust and faith. As a result, I realize that whatever I am today is due to my trust and faith in my teacher and his blessing in return.

Likewise, this makes me think of a colleague, Amchi Nel De Jong from Amsterdam, Netherlands. She was very dedicated to Rinpoche and Chagpori. When she finished her studies, she completely dedicated herself to Chagpori, supporting the development of the institute. I went to visit her in Amsterdam, during one of my tours in Europe, and I found that she lived a very simple life and was completely dedicated to her practice. All of this shows how she entrusted herself to Rinpoche as her teacher so completely and wholeheartedly.

The Purpose of a Perfect Teacher

"The purpose of adhering to the aspects of having a
perfect teacher is to learn quickly and
to become an expert."

Once we find the perfect teacher and follow them with pure intention, we will then definitely be able to achieve the goal of becoming an accomplished physician. Not only that, but by establishing this pure relationship with the teacher, our learning and progress will happen quickly. Aspiring physicians in the Tibetan tradition each have the opportunity to seek out a teacher who embodies these precious qualities, to establish a relationship with healing at its core, and to integrate these practices into their daily lives and their practice as healing agents. Hence, having the perfect teacher will meet all the student's requirements for becoming a good physician.

The Company

"Diligence with respect to one's fellow students and
colleagues is to share knowledge with friends, debate
with peers, ask questions of elders, and analyze and
retain medical teachings in the mind. One must not
succumb to laziness because it is an enemy, which
distracts the learner from studying."

Friends who encourage us to leave our studies, to go out and watch movies or go to parties, are a distraction to our study and practice. It may seem strange, but friends of this nature can actually be enemies in disguise. It is more beneficial to seek friends who support our study, who even engage in conversation and debate about these fields and can understand when we have work to do.

Here, it is very important to learn that we should not waste our precious time with company or friends who distract us from our studies. Instead, we should engage with our friends to gain more knowledge by debating, sharing, and discussing. In choosing friends, it is good to seek those who have more knowledge and experience so that they can guide us in learning. It is also good to find friends who are also engaged in study, even if they have different views, so that we can debate and seek out deeper meanings from our study.

Habituation

*"Being diligent in gaining knowledge of medicine
and its practice requires consistent mindfulness and
practice of what one has learned, either from seeing
or hearing, until it is integrated with the practice,
leaving no room for any doubt."*

Special attention must be given to the text, to the teacher, and to the environment of those around us. While we must be diligent in gaining medical knowledge and applying its practice, the final key is in maintaining awareness and retaining knowledge, so that the science of healing may be fully accomplished. When we bring awareness to our daily activities, we can learn from each circumstance that arises. All phenomena have Buddha nature and can be viewed as our teacher. This brings us to a total habituation of the healing practice, where there is no room for any doubt or sense of inferiority.

Diligence with Respect to Patients

"One is not delayed or careless while
treating the patient."

Being negligent or procrastinating could possibly inhibit the successful treatment of the patient. The physician takes every opportunity to care for the patient because they don't know when the disease may worsen or develop complications. In our busy and stressful lives, we should not neglect our patients by delaying or by being careless, even if we are attending to other patients.

"One is totally focused, as though one is balanced
atop a narrow wall, with the task of carrying a cup
of melted butter, having the consequence of death
if any is spilled."

The above metaphor is from a story about a king who gives a subject the task of carrying a cup of melted butter across a rooftop while there are dancers and musicians performing on either side. The consequence of spilling even a single drop of butter is death. For our purposes here, the subject carrying the melted butter is the physician, while the cup of melted butter is symbolic of the patient's health and life. In the story, there are also distractions around to make the task even more difficult.

This metaphor represents the imminent nature of illness and the importance of focus in medical practice. When a patient has an imbalance, it can appear to be mild or serious, but we don't know what the outcome will be, so we have to proceed carefully. We must not neglect or delay a problem because it seems mild or give very strong therapies or medicines because we think the problem is very severe. The physician needs to match the treatment with the disorder. Health and life can be very fragile, and it is important to proceed carefully, in a timely manner, with the focus on maintaining balance.

During diagnosis and treatment, the physician should be as focused as a person carrying a cup of melted butter on a rooftop. You are taking on the risk of another person's life, which is as precious as your own. It also means that the physician should not only look at the physical symptoms, but should also understand the patient's emotions, sentiments, and the underlying cause of suffering.

> *"The medication and therapies are then applied with*
> *full concentration and timeliness as if it were*
> *one's own life at stake."*

Here, the text explains the gist of the metaphor. As was mentioned above, it is very important not to neglect or ignore patients, but to apply immediate medications and therapies with full concentration, as if we were treating our own life.

SOCIAL ETHICS

> *"The Physician is an expert in societal and moral*
> *values. This includes the three aspects: social*
> *conduct, spiritual conduct, and both social*
> *and spiritual conduct."*

It is very important for the physician to have social values; just being professional is not enough. Physicians act within society and adhere to societal values. If we deeply understand our spiritual values and exhibit them in life, then people will benefit from them and develop more trust and respect.

Therefore, both social and spiritual conduct are an essential part of a physician's life.

Social Conduct

> *"First of all, one learns to be well-versed and confident in the societal norms, to engage in the compassionate care of others, and to be firm, or strict in subduing ignorance and wrong views when necessary. Having those three qualities, one's aims will be fulfilled."*

The first two qualities, adapting to societal norms and compassionately caring about others, help the physician both to avoid conflict and to benefit society. The third quality encourages the physician to uphold righteousness, keeping truth and wisdom as the primary importance. This kind of compassionate action subdues ignorance and wrong views. It may involve conflict at first but will be regarded with respect in the long run. This respect will ultimately help to fulfill the physician's purpose of always benefitting others.

Since the physician engages with society on an individual level, exhibiting any form of superiority will inhibit a physician's ability to fully connect with patients. If a physician keeps away from society, it will create differences between oneself and others. Traditionally in Tibet, the physician was considered to be a spiritual practitioner, but the physician never avoided ordinary people because of this. The work of the physician lies with people in society, so it is important to be socially sensitive.

People from all cultures have impressions and expectations about physicians, and about how people should act in general. It is not necessary to comply with people's expectations, but it is very important to maintain a genuine demeanor that people can rely upon, rather than simply to focus on superficial appearances. To me, this means being clean in body, mind, and speech. We don't dress well and bathe regularly to impress others, but rather to keep ourselves clean in order to benefit others. Similarly, we focus on benefiting others through our pure thoughts, intentions, and speech.

Dr. Tsewang Tamdin, visiting physician to His Holiness the Dalai Lama, is one of the best examples of a physician who embodies perfect social conduct in both his dedication to all his patients as well as in his work to promote and preserve Traditional Tibetan Medicine. He holds great respect for all medical practices and practitioners throughout the world.

Spiritual Conduct

"In the spiritual way of life, one becomes humble,
adaptable, and contented, and wishes only
to benefit others."

Here, we are not referring to outward religious practices such as performing rituals, reciting prayers, and visiting temples or monasteries. Nor is this a discussion about belief systems. We are looking at our state of mind.

Physicians who are skilled in spiritual conduct are neither isolated from society nor considered purely spiritual, as they are not required to commit to becoming monks, nuns, or tantric practitioners. Instead, their practice is to be humble, which means not holding themselves above or separate from others, not acting in anger, not exhibiting greed, lust, pride, or jealousy, and not indulging in laziness, apathy, or ignorance.

Spiritually skilled physicians are adaptable and learn from their mistakes. They are not discouraged by obstacles and will adapt to whatever situation presents itself. They are ready to care for others anytime and anywhere they are needed. Lastly, spiritual physicians are content with their profession of attending to suffering beings irrespective of their personal circumstances.

With all of these qualities, there is the wish to benefit others. Many physicians may have knowledge but may not have the wish to help others. A spiritually skilled physician always works to benefit other sentient beings.

Combining Social and Spiritual Conduct

"To be skilled in the combination of social and spiritual conduct, one maintains compassion for the underprivileged. The exalted ones will then fulfill their meaningful desires."

The essential point of combining societal conduct with spiritual conduct is the extension of compassion towards the poor, the diseased, and the less privileged.

Helping the poor or destitute does not exclude rich people, for they too can be poor in important areas, including health. Sometimes people are very wealthy but possess the illness of miserliness. There are many patients who have enough money to eat whatever they want, but who cannot digest anything. Some of them are materially rich but can't even get out of bed. The proverb "Health is wealth" is true. The physician will see anyone who needs to be helped and will help them without partiality.

In following these ethics, the physician will be recognized and renowned in society. The basis of this idea of being renowned is the rule of causation. Thus, helping suffering beings unconditionally (the cause), results in others help-ing you (the effect). It can appear in the professional form of superiors recognizing your efforts, or it can appear in the spiritual form of the great bodhisattvas, the kindhearted heroes, fulfilling your meaningful desires.

When we are genuinely helping suffering beings, our minds are free of considerations such as wondering how much money this will bring us or how it might help our careers. We don't expect anything in return when we help others, since that would make our actions conditioned, and those around us, including our own selves, would recognize the pretense. The physician offers pure unconditional care, and then, due to the law of causation, beneficial results may well appear within this life or the next. We don't look for them, and yet we can be assured that these positive results will happen.

> *"Having these six prerequisite qualities will bear*
> *fruit without a doubt."*

These fruits are threefold: the opportunity for spiritual prac-tice, prosperity, and true happiness. In the temporal sense of this life, this can include renown, popularity, and knowledge. However, in the spiritual realm, great bliss and liberation can be attained.

This concludes the chapter on the prerequisite qualities of the physician. We have explored three kinds of intelligence; the three stages of a compassionate heart; the six vows, two commitments, and three wisdoms of pure intention; skillful-ness with regard to body, speech, and mind; diligence towards oneself and toward others; and, finally, the social and spiri-tual conduct of being a physician.

Recommendation for Practice: Remembering We're All the Same

When neuroscience researchers studied thirteen master practitioners of Tibetan Buddhism, they discovered something amazing: as their subjects performed a simple compassion meditation, activity in the area of the brain associated with both happiness and empathy increased by as much as 800 percent. This can be an extremely healing experience. One of the subjects said this helped him to conquer his childhood panic attacks.

Do It Yourself

Yongey Mingyur Rinpoche, coauthor of *The Joy of Living,* says, "It can be enough just to think about what it is that you want—happiness, an end to suffering, etc.—and remember that everyone else in the world wants the same thing." Try this and see what happens.

"Compassion is not religious business;
it is human business. It is not luxury;
it is essential for our own peace and mental
stability. It is essential for human survival."
—His Holiness the Fourteenth Dalai Lama

Chapter 2

THE NATURE OF THE PHYSICIAN

"The nature of the Physician refers to one who fully knows each and every characteristic of the bodily constituents, the humors, the basis of disturbance, and their treatments."

To become accomplished in all of these aspects of Tibetan medicine is really quite a challenge. Traditionally in Tibet, physicians were not considered ready to practice medicine until they knew every aspect of the medical practice. As a result, there were no specialists like there are today in modern medicine with its cardiologists, nephrologists, dermatologists, psychiatrists, and such. Each physician worked with whatever illness they encountered and with whichever patient was in need.

At the same time, the physician was a spiritual practitioner whose goal was to lead others toward the ultimate relief from suffering and its cause, which is ignorance. This cannot be done by someone who is also caught in the cycle of ignorance and suffering. If you are drowning, how can you save someone else who is drowning? So, according to this profound and longstanding tradition, the physician has to combine medical knowledge with spiritual knowledge.

The first aspect of the physician's practice is to have a deep and complete knowledge of anatomy and physiology. In Traditional Tibetan Medicine, all illness arises from the imbalance, disturbance, or harm of one or more of the seven bodily constituents and the three excretions. This is called *dNod-bya* (pronounced *nod ja*), which translates as "that which is harmed." The seven bodily constituents are: nutritional essence (*Dangs-ma*), blood (*Khrag*), flesh (*Sha*), fat (*Tshil*), bone (*Rus*), bone marrow (*rKang*), and reproductive fluid (*Khu-ba*). The three excretions, also called major excretions, are: feces (*Shang*), urine (*gChin-pa*), and perspiration (*rNgul*). These are the areas of the body that are harmed in the event of a disease. The vital organs, the hollow organs, the sense organs, the reproductive organs, and the channels (which includes the systems of blood, nerves, and lymph) are all part of the constituents as well. The minor excretions, such as earwax, body oils, eye excretions, and mucus (phlegm), also fall under the major excretions. The knowledge of *dNod-bya* goes from deep and subtle to gross and intellectual. The physician must know the body inside out, and how it functions.

The second aspect is to have complete knowledge of the basis of disturbance or imbalance, *gNod-byed* (pronounced *nod-jed*), which translates as "that which harms." As stated earlier, the humors, or malfunctions, of the body are: *rLung* (wind), *mKhris-pa* (bile), and *Badkan* (phlegm). Each of these humors has five subcategories. The five winds are: the life-sustaining wind, the ascending wind, the pervasive wind, the fire-accompanying wind, and the descending wind. The five biles are: the digestive bile, the color-transforming bile, the accomplishing bile, the sight-giving bile, and the complexion-clearing bile. The five phlegms are: the supportive phlegm, the decomposing phlegm, the experiencing phlegm, the satisfying phlegm, and the connecting phlegm. Each of these subcategories facilitates the functions in the body, and all are essential for life.

Without these humors, there is no life and no sickness. The body constituents, without the humors, cannot be harmed, because they, in isolation, are without life. The physician knows the functions of the body in health and disease in a deep and complete way.

Treatment Through the Body

With thorough knowledge of the body and its functions, the physician can easily identify disease. With correct identification and diagnosis, the illness can then be accurately treated. Treatment of disease is done through balancing the bodily constituents and the bodily functions. The treatments are given through body, speech, and mind.

When using the body to treat the disease, the physician looks at and feels the body of the patient in order to make a diagnosis. Then the treatment is applied through both medications and therapies. The medications prescribed include those that pacify the disease through balancing the humors of the body, as well as those that cleanse the body of disease. Traditional Tibetan pacifying medicines are decoctions, powders, pills, medicinal butters, pastes, medicinal wines, concentrates, medicinal ashes, medicinal gems, and fresh or raw compounds. Examples of cleansing medicines are purgatives, laxatives, enemas, nasal cleanses, and eyewashes.

The therapies of Traditional Tibetan Medicine can be gentle or coarse. The gentle therapies are massage, the application of unguents, oils, powders, hot and cold compresses, water therapies, and smoke and steam inhalations. The coarse therapies are cauterization, venesection, copper cupping,

horn therapies, needle therapies, and surgical spoon therapies. Any of these treatments may be given to the patient by
the physician.

Treatment Through the Speech

The physician uses speech to investigate the nature of the disease: the patient's perception of the illness, the history of the
illness, and the symptoms. The physician uses speech wisely
to advise the patient, nurse, or caregiver on when to take the
medicines, what diet is to be followed, what is to be avoided,
and what lifestyle activities are to be adopted. The physician
also employs speech in gentle, helpful, and pleasant ways that
help soothe the patient's suffering and can guide the patient
out of ignorance, which is the cause of suffering. The physician also uses speech to heal the patient by reciting the healing mantras.

Treatment Through the Mind

The mind is engaged in the treatment through the use of
analysis and clairvoyance, in order to recognize the disease
and its appropriate treatment. The physician also uses the
mind to help relieve suffering: through a method called
Tonglen (*gTong Len*), which is a profound Buddhist practice
of exchanging one's own happiness for the suffering of others.

Tonglen (The Profound Practice of Giving and Taking)

This supreme practice is an important Buddhist practice which involves taking all illness from suffering beings
and giving all energy, goodness, and blessings to them. It
is intended to help the physician gain deeper compassion

and accumulate maximum virtuous acts, which will lead
to an enlightened state. Shantideva says in *The Way of the
Bodhisattva (Bodhicharyavatara):*

> If I do not interchange
> My happiness for others' pain,
> Enlightenment will never be attained,
> And even in samsara, joy will fly from me.

> All the joy the world contains
> Has come through wishing happiness for others
> All the misery the world contains
> Has come through wanting pleasure for oneself.

In this practice, we visualize that our own mother is sitting in
front of us, and we recollect all the good things that she has
showered upon us. Then we think of how all sentient beings
have, at one time, been our kind mother, and that each of
these beings has showered us with love, care, and support,
just like our present mother. This gives rise to great love and
appreciation for all our kind mothers.

Now we accept the suffering of others as our own suffering. All sentient beings are affected by the suffering of birth,
illness, aging, and death, which are natural processes of life.
Self-grasping and the inability to accept these natural aspects
only increase these sufferings through stress. This leads to
depression, anxiety, and many states of disease. Here we
develop our minds' capacity so that we ourselves can acknowl-
edge and receive all of the suffering of others and offer them
happiness in return.

Tonglen, the practice of giving and receiving, is performed
along with the breath. While inhaling, we visualize accepting the suffering of all sentient beings in the form of black

smoke through the nostrils. This black smoke goes directly to the core of our own self-grasping ego and is immediately transformed into bodhichitta, the mind of enlightenment. When exhaling, we visualize wholeheartedly that all of our happiness, merit, love, and prosperity is emitted as blue light pouring out of our nostrils into the hearts of all beings, easing all of their suffering. It is important to note that there is no possibility of danger or harm being done to anyone here. This intentional practice helps us to recognize the interdependence of self and other. This is the most profound use of the mind to help relieve others from suffering. As was quoted from Shantideva earlier, "All the joy the world contains has come through wishing happiness for others." Indeed, a study of toddlers that measured facial and body language, found they made the happiest expressions when they gave away their own precious treats, compared to when they themselves received treats.[1] This shows our innate nature is to experience joy and happiness through acts of generosity and compassion.

Tonglen is a sacred practice that involves spiritual rituals before it is performed and shouldn't be practiced without instruction and guidance from a teacher.

Recommendation for Practice: Being Mindful

As they go about their day, Tibetan monks practice mindfulness—being aware of all that is around them—says Yongey Mingyur Rinpoche. In a study, it was discovered that workers who practiced mindfulness for forty minutes a day had a thicker cerebral cortex, the area of the brain involved in decision-making, attention, and memory—a finding that was

---

[1] Aknin, Lara B., J. Kiley Hamlin, and Elizabeth W. Dunn. "Giving leads to happiness in young children." *PLoS One* 7.6 (2012): e39211.

even more pronounced in older meditators, since the cerebral cortex tends to thin as we age.

Do It Yourself

Mindfulness practice means being aware of your internal and external environment: sensory experiences, thoughts, and emotions. "You can do it at any time or place," says Mingyur Rinpoche. "If you're eating, for example, simply take the time to notice the color and taste and smell of your food."

"Every person has the same right as we do: to be happy and not to suffer. So let's take care of others wholeheartedly, both our friends and our enemies. This is the basis for true compassion."
—His Holiness the Fourteenth Dalai Lama

Chapter 3

THE DEFINITION OF THE PHYSICIAN

"The definition of the Physician is one who heals diseases and improves the state of the patient's well-being. One is courageous while applying the therapies upon the disease and, like a father, protects all suffering beings. Even kings will give due respect to the Physician."

This section of "The Physician Chapter" explores the various names given to a physician. The term for physician in Tibetan is *sMan-Pa* (pronounced *men-pa*). The meaning of *sMan* is "that which benefits the body and heals disease." In general, *Pa* signifies "the doer"—the one who acts or performs. This is similar to the English language suffix "-er," which also designates the doer (as "heal" becomes "healer").

Here, the use of *Pa* has two further connotations. *Pa'* is short for *dPa*, which means "courageous" or "brave." Like a brave warrior who wields his weapons to fight for a cause, the physician prescribes medicine and performs therapies with confidence and courage. *Pa* can also be *Pha*, which means "father." This is to signify the protection and care that the physician offers to patients and all sentient beings. Just as a father protects and cares for his family, the physician works for all sentient beings as though they were his own children.

Tibetan physicians are also called *Amchi*, which is a Mongolian word for physician. This is due to the Mongolian influences on Tibetan culture during the sixteenth century. Even the most well-known title for His Holiness, "Dalai Lama," is a Mongolian term which means "Ocean of Wisdom."

The physician can also be called *Lha-rJe* (pronounced *lha-je*), which literally means God King, or King of the Kings. Traditionally in Tibet, the king was considered to be like a god for his kingdom, and many were also thought to be manifestations of the bodhisattvas. The kings would determine what happened in the region, so people gave them the title, *Lha*, which means god. *rJe* means Lord, or Supreme One. It is a term that people would often use for the king. So the significance of the title, *Lha-rJe*, is that even kings would hold the physician above them as most supreme, as kings themselves were also subject to sickness and death. It is the physician who can save their lives and guide them to long life and prosperity.

Dr. Pema Dorjee writes in his book, *The Spiritual Medicine of Tibet: Heal Your Spirit, Heal Yourself*: "Historically, the greatest physicians have always been held in high regard within Tibet and accordingly been given titles such as *Menpa*, the Benefactor and Emperor of the Kings, for kings give respect to a great physician just as they would to an Emperor. Indeed, physicians acquire respect and renown, not through any form of advertising or a long list of qualifications but through their level of sensitivity shown towards the patient and the quality of their compassion, selflessness, and innate wisdom, combined with a pure focus on the source of all healing, the Medicine Buddha.

Recommendation for Practice: Sitting Up Straight

Before any meditation, Tibetan monks straighten their spines by sitting or standing with their shoulders back—and for good reason: research shows much of the brain's energy comes from nerves in the spinal cord. "And the better your posture, the more efficiently the spinal neurons can fire, and the more of your brainpower you can access," explains chiropractor Richard Weinstein, D.C.

Do It Yourself
Sit with a straight spine, lifting the top of your head, which tucks the chin slightly. Gently draw your shoulders back and down. Try maintaining this posture, and your awareness of it, when you read the next chapter, and see what happens.

"A good life does not mean just good food, good clothes, and good shelter. These are not sufficient. A good motivation is what is needed: compassion without dogmatism, without complicated philosophy; just understanding that others are human brothers and sisters and respecting their rights and human dignity."
—His Holiness the Fourteenth Dalai Lama

Chapter 4

CLASSIFICATION OF THE PHYSICIAN

"The three classifications of Physicians are:
supreme, extraordinary, and general."

THE SUPREME PHYSICIAN

"The supreme Physician is the highest Physician who
can dispel the causational three mental poisons and
the resultant diseases."

The *rGyud-bZhi* describes dispelling the cause and result of the three mental poisons. The ultimate cause of these mental poisons—attachment, aversion, and delusion—is ignorance. The fruits of these mental poisons are the imbalanced three humors—*rLung* (wind), *mKhris-pa* (bile), and *Badkan* (phlegm).

When a supreme physician completely dispels all suffering and its qualities, what then remains is complete enlightenment or liberation. Since disease results from the ultimate cause of ignorance, which takes the form of the three poisons, then it follows that to be free of disease means to be completely free of ignorance. The path to accomplishing this is through the union of compassion and wisdom.

The supreme physician who can dispel the cause and result of the mental poisons is the Unsurpassed Supreme One, a manifestation of the Medicine Buddha. In our lineage, there are some great sages who have achieved this: Jivaka Kumara, Yuthog Yonten Gonpo, Desi Sangye Gyatso, and Khenrab Norbu are all profound examples. These great physicians are revered and emulated by all Tibetan physicians. To become the unsurpassed supreme physician is the goal of all Tibetan physicians.

THE EXTRAORDINARY PHYSICIAN

"The extraordinary, venerable Physician is one who has clairvoyance, compassion, and the truthful and righteous nature of a great sage."

The extraordinary physician has three great qualities. The first is a clairvoyant mind, which, in the application of medicine, understands the patient's nature, senses, and dormant signs of imbalances. As a deep-minded aspect of intelligence, clairvoyance refers to heightened awareness. There are generally considered to be six types of clairvoyance: divine seeing, divine hearing, knowledge of others' thoughts and emotions, knowledge of miracles, knowledge of past and future, and knowledge of the decay and destruction of the passions in order to purify the body and mind. The development of this heightened awareness is achieved through practice, supplications, and meditation.

To give an example of clear knowledge, I would again like to refer to my teacher. When I was practicing in Darjeeling, Dr. Trogawa Rinpoche was invited by his friend's mother to diagnose her when she came down with a sudden illness. Rinpoche felt her pulse and, through his clairvoyance, predicted that what she felt was related to the arrival of her son the next day. She was surprised to hear that her son was coming without informing her. The next day, upon his arrival, her illness subsided. Here, Rinpoche was able to clearly see the cause of the problem, even though it was very subtle. This is an example of being skilled in the art of reading the seven wonder pulses.

The second aspect of the extraordinary physician is having great compassion and love for all sentient beings. Having this love motivates the extraordinary physician to work selflessly for others. When we dedicate ourselves completely to helping others, it is often felt and experienced by them, as in the example given earlier of patients stating that they felt better just by being in the presence of Dr. Trogawa Rinpoche.

The last aspect is that the extraordinary physician has the quality of a sage. As in other traditions, the sage is truthful and righteous. It takes wisdom to abide in truth and not succumb to personal aversions and attractions. Men-Tsee-Khang put this very beautifully in their translation of *The Root Tantra and Explanatory Tantra*: "...they [the extraordinary physicians] righteously rectify the defects of their body, speech, and mind and harmonize all the imbalances of others."

I have encountered some extraordinary physicians in my life, including my teacher, the late Dr. Trogawa Rinpoche, and the late Dr. Tenzin Choedrak, senior personal physician to His Holiness the Fourteenth Dalai Lama. These great physicians have influenced people with their patience, affection, compassion, and wisdom.

When I was working at the Chagpori Tibetan Medical Clinic, there was a monk who became paralyzed. He consulted a Lama who then performed a divination for him. The divination revealed that he should seek the treatment of

Dr. Trogawa Rinpoche. The monk requested that Rinpoche come to see him for treatment. During that time, Rinpoche was at a retreat, so I was sent to analyze the patient's pulse and urine. The patient was unable to speak or move his limbs. I reported my findings to Rinpoche, who then had an idea about how to treat the monk. Rinpoche explained to me that the monk's paralysis was not only caused by a nerve disorder but was also due to spirit obstacles. He prescribed a treatment of medications that could help to remove these obstacles, and over time, the monk recovered from the paralysis. A neurologist who was earlier treating the monk was very surprised by his unlikely recovery.

I also observed that Dr. Tenzin Choedrak—despite being the personal physician to His Holiness the Fourteenth Dalai Lama—was enthusiastic, full of affection, selfless, and happy to see any patient that came to him. This showed his great compassion and humility. He was always available to see any patient, regardless of whether there was an appointment or not. He was also humble and generous.

I was also fortunate to receive the transmission of the *rGyud-bZhi* from Dr. Choedrak while working at Men-Tsee-Khang in Dharamsala. At the time, he must have been in his seventies. He had such clarity in knowing the text that hearing him give the transmission flawlessly was like listening to Yuthog Yonten Gonpo himself.

THE GENERAL PHYSICIAN

"The general Physician is of a royal lineage, has learned from a qualified physician, or has gained practical experience from a teacher. These lineages of Physicians are friends of all suffering beings."

These classifications of the general physician show how the training of a Tibetan physician is acquired. The first method is the method of the royal lineage, which is the one that has been passed down since the first royal physician in Tibet, Dung gi Thor Chog (Dungi Thorchog). From him, the tradition of medicine was handed down from teacher to student, mostly within the same family.

This lineage was passed down to Yuthog Yonten Gonpo the Younger, a master physician who recompiled the medical text, the *rGyud-bZhi*, into its present form. He was also a realized master who turned the spiritual practice of the physician into a sublime practice. This is known as the Yuthog Nyingthig (Yuthog Heart Essence Practice). It is a complete spiritual practice that nearly all Tibetan physicians have been following since his time. In Tibet, it was said that the physician was considered to be incomplete without receiving this practice, and that it is only through receiving the transmission, empowerment, and explanation of it that one is able to carry on the lineage.

These three—empowerment, *Wang (dBang)*; transmission, *Loong (Lung)*; and explanation, *Tri ('Khrid)*—are essential aspects to all Vajrayana Buddhist practices. The first is the empowerment, when the teacher gives the student the initiation, experience, or feeling of the spiritual practice. The second is the transmission of the practice, in which the teacher reads the text and relates the basic instructions. The third, the explanation, is when the teacher explains the outer, inner, and secret meanings of the practice. All three of these are necessary for a complete practice.

These teachings and practices have been passed down for many generations and are continuing in modern times. It is very important to follow all of the practices that we have received from our teachers. This is how lineages and spiritual practices continue.

The second method of becoming a physician is through academic study with a qualified physician or scholar. This is how people in medical colleges learn. To be qualified, the teacher has to have heard, read, and seen all the theoretical aspects of the medical practice. The qualified teacher also needs to have experience in the application of medicine. With both the textual knowledge and experiential knowledge, the physician is then qualified to pass on the teachings.

The final method is attaining medical experience through working with a master as an apprentice. The whole system of medicine is experiential in essence, and the student can become adept by working with a master. The knowledge of the anatomy of the body can be shown and felt. The knowledge of diagnosis has to come through seeing, touching, and questioning. And the application of treatments of a disease can be learned by paying close attention to what a teacher says and does. Then, helping the teacher in the actual treatment of patients will accustom the student to the practice. In this way, it is possible to become a beneficial physician.

As stated above, by learning through any of these three methods—the royal lineage, studying with a qualified teacher, or gaining experience with a master—the student becomes a friend to all sentient beings. This means that all of these methods can make us physicians suitable to benefit others through the medical practice.

"But those who, out of desire, immediately assume the practice of healing without learning well, are destroyers of life."

This statement emphasizes the necessity of being learned in the study and practice of medicine before beginning to treat patients. Those who take short courses and claim to be physicians because of their desire for material wealth or recognition will inevitably make mistakes and cause harm to their patients. In this way, they also ruin the tradition of the medical lineage, and thus become destroyers of life.

"The classifications can also be considered in terms of superior and inferior Physicians."

There are two classifications: one is the superior physician and the other is the inferior physician.

The Superior Physician

"The superior Physician is of a genuine lineage, intelligent, and fully devoted to the practice; clearly knows the meaning of the medical theories; has received the secret instructions; and is accurate in giving therapies. The Physician is well-experienced, has a habit of performing spiritual practices, and avoids mundane desires. They are humble, and skillful in manufacturing medicines and medical instruments, and have limitless compassion for all suffering beings. They do not lose focus, and [they] think of others' welfare as their own purpose. Therefore, a superior Physician is not ignorant of any of the healing therapies and is the sole protector of all sentient beings. They are the prince lineage holder of the numerous scholars and sages. It is said that this is the incarnation of the great healer, the Medicine Buddha."

This genuine lineage in Traditional Tibetan Medicine comes down from the historical Buddha and many other great historical sages who were physicians. However, this quality can come from any genuine lineage, according to "The Root Tantra" of the *rGyud-bZhi*, as the Medicine Buddha gave his teaching to many great ones, sages, nonBuddhists, and Buddhists. Each of these disciples understood the teachings in their own language. In other words, there are as many branches of healing as there are cultures in the world, and each was born out of the wisdom of healing. The basic qualities of healing and the basic nature of the healer are transmitted through each of these lineages.

As noted previously, intelligence refers to the three qualities of broad-mindedness, stable-mindedness, and deep-mindedness. Intelligence also applies to the sense of being able to differentiate between right and wrong. The physician should understand fully the difference between right and wrong actions of body, speech, and mind in order to remain balanced while treating patients.

Devotion to the practice is the pure intention of *Dam-Tshig*, which is commitment to both practice and lineage. There are three aspects to this, as was explored in the section on pure intention: the vows, the commitments, and the wisdoms. The superior physician displays purity in all these aspects.

Knowing the medical theories comes from hearing, seeing, and reading the medical texts and commentaries. These theories are then explained, and practical instructions are given. The physician is guided in realizing the secrets of the body, disease, and treatments by a qualified expert.

The superior physician is fully accustomed to the practice of helping suffering beings. This comes from being developed in the spiritual practice of realizing the nature of all phenomena, and keeping all actions of body, speech, and mind compassionate. By being humble, the physician abandons desire and greed. This is accomplished by taming the three gates of the body, speech, and mind.

Being skilled in compounding and prescribing medicines refers to knowing the tastes, powers, qualities, and post-digestive effects of the ingredients. The superior physician knows which types of compounds apply to specific diseases, and whether they should be pacifying or cleansing with internal or external applications.

A superior physician skilled in the therapies knows the medical instruments so well that they have become easy to use. The instrument should be adapted to the hand of the user and the therapy being performed. Each medical instrument is perfectly proportioned for the practitioner and its components are chosen for optimizing the medicinal effect.

Limitless compassion and love for all sentient beings is gained through practice. The superior physician has boundless energy to help poor and suffering sentient beings. This is the main intent of the compassionate heart.

The superior physician does not lose focus or get distracted from thinking about others' welfare. Even an instant of distraction can be enough to make a mistake in treating a disease.

For this reason, helping others is valued more highly than helping our own selves—ultimately, happiness is dependent on the happiness of others. Thus, we take great joy in seeing patients and other sentient beings become free from suffering.

This gives the physician motivation to completely learn all healing therapies in both theory and in practice. The therapies are not applied randomly or with too much enthusiasm, but according to the need. The superior physician, having received all the secret transmissions from the master, knows how to apply the therapies at the right time and right place.

The physician takes on the role of being the sole protector of all sentient beings, which gives a drive and determination to work tirelessly. Just as in the pure intention section of the prerequisite qualities, which spoke of the two commitments, this relates to the lineage-holding physician committed to being a Dharma protector. Here, the view of the physician is amplified into being the ultimate protector.

Having all of these qualities, the superior physician is noble in upholding the lineage of the great scholars and sages of the past such as Jivaka Kumara, Yuthog Yonten Gonpo, Desi Sangye Gyatso, Khenrab Norbu, and many more.

A present-day example of a superior physician is Dr. Yeshe Dondhen, a senior practitioner and former personal physician to the Fourteenth Dalai Lama. He was the founder and first teacher at Men-Tsee-Khang in Dharamsala, India. In 2018 he was honored by the Indian president and received the highest civilian award, the Padma Shree, for his contribution to healing countless patients especially ones diagnosed with cancer. He dedicated his life to treating his patients. He retired at the age of ninety-two in April 2019 and peacefully passed away seven months later.

With all of these supreme qualities, the superior physician is none other than the Medicine Buddha, himself. Each person has Buddha nature within themselves, and when this nature is directed towards healing and is complete, with all the qualities of the superior physician, this is the attainment of the state of Medicine Buddha, the great healer, the Medicine King.

The Inferior Physician

"An inferior Physician is incomplete in the qualities
of the superior Physician."

This simply means that if the qualities of the superior physician are not present, then the physician is considered inferior.

"A Physician without a lineage is like a fox ruling
the kingdom; they will not be honored or
respected by anyone."

The metaphor here is that a fox is trying to rule the kingdom when the lion is the real king. Here, the physician without a lineage is the fox, while the lineage-holder is the lion. This deception may work in the beginning, but eventually, people will recognize the shortcomings of the impostor.

Thus, a physician without an authentic lineage who continues to treat patients is like a fox trying to rule the kingdom.

"A Physician who does not know the meaning
of the text is like pointing out an object to a blind
person. The disease types and healing methods
are not understood."

The physician who does not understand the medical texts will not be able to apply the medical theory in practice. The physician is then blind to the medical practice. The metaphor is that the blind person would not be able to identify any object, even if it were pointed out. Similarly, an inferior physician cannot identify particular diseases or differentiate any of the treatments.

Thus, a physician who does not know the meaning of the medical text is as effective as showing an object to the blind.

"A Physician without the experience of seeing is like someone going down an unknown path; there will be doubt in recognizing symptoms and corresponding treatments."

When traveling down an unknown path or road, one doesn't know where it will turn or what obstacles will appear. In the same way, if a physician has not seen and experienced the medical theories in practice, then there will be doubt, especially concerning the signs and symptoms of disorders. There are many symptoms that can look similar but have different qualities. The physician must be adept at determining the cause of a disease in order to affect a cure, which is done through subtle awareness and analysis developed from experience.

Thus, the inexperienced physician is like a doubtful traveler, traversing an unfamiliar path.

"A Physician who does not know the diagnostic methods is like someone roaming around a foreign place without familiar people; not a single disease will be recognized."

As any traveler knows, the best way to see a place is with someone who knows it well. If we have a friend, relative, or guide who can show us the way to the places we wish to visit, it makes for less confusion and reduces the chances of getting lost. The physician who does not know the diagnostic methods is like a traveler wandering in a foreign land without any guide. Without knowing the diagnostic methods, we will not be able to recognize a single disorder.

Thus, the physician who lacks skill in diagnostic methods is like a foreign traveler without a friend or guide.

"A Physician who does not know the pulse or urine analysis is like a spy who does not know espionage. Differentiation of hot and cold diseases will not be known."

What is the work of a spy? The most important job for a spy is collecting information. It is the same for the physician regarding the diagnostic techniques of pulse diagnosis and urine analysis. The patient will come with many signs, symptoms, lifestyle activities, and dietary habits, but the physician feels the pulse and looks at the urine to check the nature of the disease. The most essential aspect in diagnosis is determining whether the nature of the disease is hot or cold. If the physician gets this correct, then there will not be any countereffects from the medicines and treatments given. On the other hand, if it is wrong, then the physician's work, which is supposed to help the patient, will actually cause harm.

Thus, a physician who does not know pulse reading and urine analysis is like a spy who does not know how to recognize valuable information.

"A Physician who cannot speak with confidence (make a prognosis) is like a leader who does not know how to give orders. This will belittle oneself and lead to a bad reputation."

The term "prognosis" here relates to announcing how the disease will progress or be pacified, and whether the patient will live or die. These types of announcements must be made carefully and accurately in order to build trust and faith with the patient. If the physician cannot predict the outcome of the disease and is ignorant of how to skillfully speak with the patient, then the reputation of the physician will suffer. Just as a leader unskillful at speaking will lose the respect and confidence of the people, similarly, a physician unable to make a prognosis confidently will also lose the respect and confidence of the patients.

Thus, a physician who does not know how to make a prognosis is like a leader who cannot speak skillfully, as the situation demands.

> *"A Physician who does not know the treatment*
> *methods is like someone attempting to hit a target*
> *in the dark. The remedy will not reach*
> *the disease."*

If someone tries to shoot an arrow in a dark place, how likely will they succeed in hitting the target? If a physician knows the treatment methods like diet, lifestyle, medications, and therapies completely, then the physician will be able to affect a cure or at least benefit the patient. In that case, the response towards the treatment will be good, and some relief will come to the patient. If a physician does not know the treatments and gives wrong medicines, then it will only complicate the disease and cause harm in the long run.

Thus, a physician who does not know how to treat a disease is like someone who shoots at a target in the dark.

> *"A Physician who does not know dietary and lifestyle*
> *behaviors is like a leader whose constituency has*
> *turned into enemies. Diseases will gain strength and*
> *the body will deteriorate."*

If there is a mutiny within the kingdom and even the king's friends turn against him, then his rule will falter and all may be ruined. Not knowing correct diet and lifestyle recommendations can be like this. The disease can become aggravated and the bodily constituents can deteriorate from consuming the wrong diet and following harmful lifestyle activities. These two factors are the means by which we get our physical strength and immunity and are the main immediate conditions of disease.

It is beneficial for the physician to explore the patient's diet and to observe whether lifestyle activities, such as sleeping, working, socializing, thinking, bathing, and exercising, have been harmful or beneficial. This will help the physician know the cause of the problem. In advising the patient on diet and what the patient should consume and what they should avoid, the physician addresses tastes and potencies, the proper and improper combinations of ingredients, and the timing and quantity of intake of food and drinks.

For lifestyle activities, the physician knows which activities cause stress, which cause deterioration and weakness, and which aggravate illness. The seasonal effects of diet and lifestyle are equally important. Moreover, avoiding the suppression of natural functions of the body will prevent ailments from arising. When advising the patient, the physician considers all of these factors, in order not to cause further harm to the body or aggravate the disease.

Thus, a physician who does not have knowledge about diet and lifestyle is like a king who turns his own kingdom into an enemy.

> "A Physician who does not know the administration of pacifying compounds is like a farmer who does not know farming. The disease will aggravate from deficient, excess, and wrong administration."

A farmer must know about a plant's need for water and fertilizer, how to germinate seeds, and about environmental and climatic conditions—in short, how to tend the plants towards a full harvest. Similarly, a physician must know what medicinal ingredients are necessary for the disease at hand, what type of compound will benefit the disease, and what time to prescribe the medicine according to the nature of the disease and its accumulating, aggravating, and pacifying times.

The physician also has to understand the intensity of the disease in order to match the treatment with the disease. If a physician treats a fever with strong medicine to pacify the heat when the fever is actually mild, then a cold disorder can develop. Likewise, if the fever is strong and the physician prescribes mild medicine, then the fever will not come down and could become chronic. Lastly, if the physician sees a hidden fever as a cold-related problem because the patient is feeling tired and has a low appetite, and prescribes warming medicines, then the fever could increase and even become fatal. As can be seen, this knowledge of the correct technique for administering medicine is very important.

Thus, a physician who does not know how to compound a pacifying medicine is like a farmer who does not know farming.

"A Physician who does not know the actions of cleansing therapies is like someone pouring water onto a sand dune. The disease and the bodily constituents will be spoiled."

When water is poured onto a sand dune, the sand and water will mix and the hill will collapse. Similarly, when the physician is applying the various cleansing techniques (oil therapies, emesis, purgation, laxatives, enemas, nasal cleanses, eyewashes, and channel-cleansing techniques), it is very important to match the therapy to the disease that it is supposed to benefit. The physician must perform the cleansing at a particular time, as timing is an important factor in the effectiveness of these therapies. A disease that has spread must first be collected and removed from the appropriate location. Knowledge of timing and of the appropriate therapy is essential. If, for example, one were to give a vomiting therapy to someone with a *rLung* (wind) disease, not only would *rLung* aggravate, but the stomach might also develop a problem.

Thus, a physician who does not know cleansing therapy is like someone pouring water onto a sand dune.

> *"A Physician who is without medicine and medical instruments is like a brave warrior without any weapons. One cannot vanquish the advancing enemy. The strength of the disease will therefore be undefeatable."*

Just like weapons are important to a warrior in battle, medicines and medical instruments are essential for the physician to pacify or expel the disease.

There are a few miscellaneous diseases that can be alleviated by observing a beneficial diet and lifestyle, but the majority of diseases require some intervention, like medicine and therapies, to be cured. For this, it is necessary for the physician to keep medicines and instruments available for when they are needed.

Thus, a physician without medicines and medical instruments is like a warrior without any weapons.

> *"The Physician who does not know the venesection and cauterization techniques is like a thief finding*

one's way in an unknown house. One will be
mistaken in dealing with the disease
and its therapies."

The thief who knows a house and where the jewels are kept will be successful in the theft. If the thief has no prior knowledge of the house, he will roam around looking for something to steal, and may not find anything. Likewise, the physician who does not know the channel points of venesection or the secret points of cauterization will have no impact on the targeted disease. Similarly, if the physician does not know the proper techniques of applying the therapy, they will not completely heal the problem. For example, the physician has to know the exact points on which to perform the venesection, how much blood to let, how frequently it is to be let, and the most beneficial time to perform the venesection. The same applies for cauterization and moxabustion. If a physician heats the point but does not give the amount of heat to match the disease in the correct points, then the disease will not be completely dispelled. This is true for any type of surgery or other invasive therapies, including other traditional medical systems.

Thus, a physician who does not know about venesection and cauterization is like a thief finding their way in an unknown house.

"Therefore, an inferior Physician has misconceptions
about the healing knowledge and will give all
the wrong treatments. This is like the Lord of
Death holding a noose as a weapon in the guise
of a Physician holding medical instruments. The
treatment could have fatal effects. It is as though
the patient is caught in the noose of the Lord of

Death. It is not beneficial to keep relations with such
imposters, as they will ruin their patients."

The twelve defects of the inferior physician, as stated above, will result in misapprehension of all medical theories of the body, disease, diagnosis, and treatment. As a result, the patient may be harmed. Inferior physicians are actually destroyers of life rather than preservers of life. The demon of the Lord of Death is well known in Tibetan culture and religion. The Lord of Death escorts beings from this life into the *bardo*, the intermediate state. This demon is an emissary of the Lord of Death, who does evil and can even take life before the lifespan is exhausted. So the inferior physician is like a demon because their malfeasance could cause the patient to die before their lifespan is over.

The inferior physician is someone who tries to practice medicine without completing their medical studies and the associated clinical or practical experience. Those who take short-term courses and then practice medicine tend to become inferior physicians. Such physicians ruin the reputation of the medical practice. Maintaining relations with them will spoil one's reputation and cause much harm to those treated by them.

Recommendation for Practice: Listening to Bells

Many Tibetan prayers begin and end with the sound of bells called *tingsha*, a pair of small cymbals attached by a string. "They're used to refresh and open the mind, and since they're made by hand, no two are alike," says meditation teacher Steven Sashen. When they're struck, each of the two discs rings at a slightly different frequency. "Studies show that when you hear two different frequencies at once, your brain registers a frequency equal to the difference between the two," Sashen explains.

Do It Yourself

If you have the chance to use *tingsha* for this practice, by all means, do. Otherwise, you can take the sounds that already exist around you as objects for sound meditation. Close your eyes and be aware of any sound you hear. Do not focus on the origin or object creating the sound, but rather focus on the sensation of hearing itself. If you hear two or more sounds, try to listen to the multiple sounds with equal attention. Allow this to be an opportunity for meditation.

"The purpose of our life needs to be positive. We weren't born with the purpose of causing trouble or harming others. For our life to be of value, I think we must develop basic good human qualities— warmth, kindness, and compassion. Then our life becomes meaningful and more peaceful—happier." —His Holiness the Fourteenth Dalai Lama

Chapter 5

THE FUNCTIONS OF
THE PHYSICIAN

"The Physician's functions are two-fold:
general and specific."

This particular chapter is about the actual work of the physician. The day-to-day, general functions of the physician's body, speech, and mind are covered in the first section. The second section focuses on the specific functions of the view, meditation, and behavior of the physician. This section explores the inner perspective: the building of positive habits and the importance of being balanced in our approach as a physician.

THE GENERAL FUNCTIONS

"The general function of a Physician involves
devoting the body, speech, and mind towards the
well-being of the patients."

The three gates of the body, speech, and mind are important tools a physician can use to treat the patient. The addition of the term "devotion" implies the wholeheartedness with which physicians are encouraged to use their body, speech, and mind to benefit others.

Functions of the Physician's Body

"With regard to the body, the Physician accumulates all medicines and medical instruments; each of them relating to the patients' treatments."

The main function of the physician's body is to collect, administer, and apply medicines and therapeutics. The physician keeps the patient's well-being in mind while doing so. This means that the physician knows what diseases are to be treated and prepares the medicines and therapeutic instruments accordingly.

Traditionally, Tibetan physicians and their assistants or students would compound their own medicines and make their own instruments. They would collect the ingredients at the appropriate time of the year: shoots and flowers in the spring; bark, leaves, some flowers, and fruits in the summer; some fruits, roots, and seeds in the autumn. Then, the physicians would compound the medicines according to the diseases that needed to be treated. These days, the majority of Tibetan physicians use medicinal compounds that are standardized as per the Tibetan medical texts. These compounds are usually made in advance and kept ready for patients.

Of course, it is still relevant for the physician to consider specific patient needs while dispensing medicines. My practice is in Bangalore, and the common ailments I treat are allergies, arthritis, diabetes, migraines, kidney diseases, cancer, and so on. Therefore, it is very important for me to keep at hand the medicines needed to heal these illnesses, along with other medicines and medical instruments. Without these medicines, I would be handicapped in my medical practice. It's equally important to keep at hand other medicines and tools that will inspire confidence in the treatment and in the physician.

Another action of the body is maintenance of the physician's health, which is important as the physician needs to be ready at any time in order to serve their patients. The physical aspects of the body must be maintained as well. The hands should be soft and sensitive so that the physician can accurately feel the pulse and palpate the body. The hands should also be flexible and dexterous so that the fine work of collecting and making the medicines can be performed well, and therapeutic instruments can be made and wielded with accuracy. This is achieved through physical experience and awareness.

Functions of the Physician's Speech

"In the actions of speech, one speaks prognostic words with the confidence of blowing a conch-trumpet in the marketplace only when one thoroughly knows the diagnosis and treatment of a disorder. Physicians are able to offer a guarantee to the patient if a recovery is possible, or predict the time of death if it is not possible to heal. If unsure of the outcome, one speaks as if having a snake's tongue, and depends on two possibilities. The Physician chooses the one that is favorable."

The most important prognosis a physician can make is announcing whether the disease is treatable or not. If the physician can accurately make this prognosis it will instill trust in the patient and give the physician renown. There are other prognostications, apart from declaring life or death, such as announcing the name of an illness and the time required to cure it. During pregnancy there are questions as to whether or not the labor will have complications. There are also many ways to determine the time of death if the disease is untreatable, which, if the situation demands, can also be announced. These different types of prognoses can be made with confidence if we have deep knowledge.

If we are unsure, then we should speak very carefully, conveying both the possibility of success in treatment and also the possibility that the disease might be untreatable. This is what is meant by speaking with a snake's tongue. It is not about the physician trying to deceive the patient or about the physician being cunning. Here, speaking with a snake's tongue, which is forked, means that when we speak, we don't make clear announcements about prognosis because treatment outcomes are also dependent on karma, luck, and merit. For example, the physician might say, "You may survive if you or your family do spiritual practices like chanting, prostration, rituals, and such, which may change your karma and merit. But if you neglect this problem, or if some other obstacle arises, then spiritual practice may not help you."

Next, the physician monitors the course of treatment to see whether the disease is more likely to be cured or whether it is more likely that the patient will die. The physician looks at how the patient responds to a treatment. If there is an improvement within a short time, the physician may see the possibility of survival. However, if the disease continues to progress in spite of the treatment, then the physician sees that the patient may not survive and announces this.

The physician does this carefully so as not to disturb the patient unnecessarily. In this world, there are so many factors that cause stress; if we can say something that evokes a mental state of peace, then why not do so? At the same time, if death is imminent, it is also the physician's responsibility to help the patient prepare for a peaceful death. The physician skillfully conveys to the patient, and possibly the family, the impermanence of life and helps them recall their spiritual practices and good deeds. For optimum positive impact, the physician's speech is soft, gentle, and truthful. Here, it is so important for the patient to be able to benefit from every word the physician offers.

Other Functions of Speech

"Furthermore, the functions of speech are: to clearly paraphrase a patient's own feelings, to follow the state of the mind's resolve, and to not reject the possible outcomes that exist; it is better to avoid such difficult and unreliable predictions."

This section gives exact instructions about how to communicate with the patient. I have found this especially important because patients need to be met where they are. It does not help if we speak from a place of superiority. Instead, it is helpful to encourage self-awareness and confidence in the treatment prescribed, and to offer knowledge of how diet and lifestyle can be both beneficial and harmful.

Paraphrasing a Patient's Own Feelings (Agreeing with the Patient's Opinion)

"Firstly, make it clear when the diagnosis and patient's suspicion are similar. If the patient claims indigestion, and the Physician's diagnosis is in agreement, then the Physician should state so clearly."

This is the most ideal situation because the patient's suspicion and the physician's findings through the diagnosis match. The physician can speak frankly and directly.

Follow the State of the Mind's Resolve

> *"Secondly, the patient may have the feeling of being*
> *poisoned, but the diagnosis shows another cause.*
> *Do not announce the contradiction, but follow*
> *the patient's resolve, and treat the disease*
> *as it actually is."*

In this case, the physician does not openly contradict the patient. Patients can be cured of indigestion even if they think the cause is poison. It is the patient that suffers, and they have the right to harbor their own thoughts about the cause of the illness. The patient's opinion is valued as much as the physician's, but this does not mean that the physician will treat the disease only according to the patient's ideas and thoughts. Instead, the physician treats the disease as it actually is, without challenging the patient's perspective.

In this way, the patient can be cured of a temporary illness quickly and the physician will achieve renown for being adept. I have had experiences where this has been useful. For example, when a patient comes to me with joint pain, I may prescribe treatment based on a *rLung* (wind) disorder instead of prescribing medicine specifically intended for joint health. In some instances, the underlying cause of joint pain is a *rLung* disorder, which is related to stress and emotions, and enters the body through the bones and joints. Rather than treating the presenting symptoms, the physician identifies and treats the actual cause of the disturbance. At the conclusion of the treatment, not only is the patient free from joint pain, but they also feel the benefits of reduced stress. Traditionally, this is how the physician achieves distinction in their work. In the past, there was no media or telecommunications, so renown for a physician only came through word of mouth.

We may question the wisdom of this approach, wondering what happens if the patient later finds out that the physician did not state the correct diagnosis immediately. The simple answer is that the physician does not reside in falsehoods but uses skillful means to agree with the patient while treating the true disease. If the disease is treated correctly, then the patient will be happy to be relieved of suffering and will also respect the physician. At this point, the physician can explain that it is the cause of the illness that Traditional Tibetan Medicine treats, not the symptoms.

Complicated Predictions

"Thirdly, in the cases of surviving or dying, and the disease being a high versus low risk to the patient's life, all are dependent on luck, karma, and merit of both the patient and the Physician. The patient's recovery is also dependent on the conditions of the patient's diet and lifestyle. Due to these factors, it is difficult to make clear predictions about whether one will die or survive. In such conditions, announce that it is a serious problem but that healing is possible, or if it seems not to be so serious, warn the patient to take precautions to protect their health and life."

This is actually the case in most patients. The outcome of life is very difficult to predict. The factors of luck, karma, and merit are complex Buddhist concepts that have great influence on life. "Luck" is a term that is used in many, if not all cultures. In Tibetan, it is called *rLung-rTa* (pronounced *loong-ta*) and means "wind horse." It is like the randomness of fate or destiny, and is closely related to karma and merit, but is often used in terms of prosperity or fortune. Avoiding an accident can be called lucky and getting in a minor accident with severe results can be called unlucky. If a patient has a cold, and then gets caught in a bad snowstorm, this would be considered unlucky as it would severely aggravate the problem.

Karma is the law of causation. The Newtonian law, "To every action there is an equal and opposite reaction," is very similar to this concept. The law of causation states that for each phenomenon there is a cause that relates to the nature of that phenomenon. Karma can be directly translated as action. A karmic effect results from an earlier action. This can be from a past life or the present one. There is a Buddhist saying that explains karma in this way: "Whatever I am now is because of my past actions, and whatever I am in the future, will be because of my present actions." It's important to know that karma is not fate or a predetermined destiny; it is simply the principle of cause and effect. Karma can be easily changed by changing our actions.

Karma plays an important role in health and disease. According to Traditional Tibetan Medicine, one quarter of all illnesses are considered to be caused by karma. There are diseases caused by the karmas of this life, by the karmas of past lives, and by a combination of both. The physician can identify these disorders as a result of their spiritual development. Karmic disorders manifest as diseases that are usually not so serious, but they often remain untreatable despite the many available advanced technologies and treatments. According to Tibetan medicine, these karmic disorders require spiritual treatments such as performing rituals, chanting mantras, prostrating, and circumambulating around holy places, and practicing generosity through charity or other beneficial services. All of these spiritual practices can change the course of karmic disorders, along with the support of medical treatments.

Another aspect of karma that moves beyond the individual level is collective karma. This kind of karma occurs between people, and within families and whole societies. Some Tibetans believe that the Chinese invasion of Tibet was due to collective negative karma. But sometimes these seemingly bad karmic experiences also bring prosperity. Despite the eventual loss of the Tibetan homeland and the widespread devastation that occurred, not only has Tibetan culture survived, but in the ensuing diaspora its rich cultural and spiritual practices have been shared with the world. His Holiness continues to remind his fellow Tibetans of this more positive perspective.

Merit is gained through beneficial actions that help other beings. This means engaging in virtuous activities and avoiding non-virtuous ones. We also gain merit from engaging in spiritual activities. An example of good merit would be His Holiness the Fourteenth Dalai Lama, who came from a peasant family and rose to become Tibet's spiritual, political, and globally-acclaimed leader. An example of lacking merit would be someone who comes into great wealth or opportunity but lacks the merit to enjoy and benefit from the prosperity.

The final condition that determines the outcome of the physician's treatment is the patient's diet and lifestyle, and the patient's willingness to comply with the physician's advice. If someone pours water on a fire while another person pours kerosene, it is very difficult to put the fire out. Similarly, if the physician tries to cure an ailment with medicine and therapies while the patient follows a diet and behaves in ways that aggravates the problem, it becomes very difficult to cure the disease.

All of these factors are dependent on both the patient and the physician. They both need to have luck, karma, merit, and the right state of mind in order to cure the illness. When any of these factors are deficient, then the disease may not be cured and may, in fact, become fatal. Due to all these factors, making an accurate prognosis can be very difficult, and often it is better to avoid making such definitive statements.

I tell most of my patients who say that I have cured their disease that it is not possible to make a sound by clapping with one hand, and similarly, it is not possible to cure a disease only through medical treatment. Patients have an equal responsibility to follow a healthy diet, lifestyle, positive thinking, and spiritual practice.

If we recognize that the disease is serious but are not sure whether the patient will die from it, then it is best to say that it is a serious problem, but there is a possibility of a cure. Here, we help the patient with treatment and we also suggest spiritual practices, which can overcome disorders and obstacles.

If we see that the problem is not so serious, we might be inclined to say that the problem could become worse, and that the patient should take precautions to avoid that from happening. Here, the aim is to maintain their health and not to make the disease worse.

> *"Yet again it is important to follow the socially accepted norms and customs while making predictions."*

A skillful physician considers what the patient can accept based on their cultural beliefs and social norms. An example of this would be the differences found in treating Western patients versus treating patients from the East. We all know that stress, negativity, and depression are major factors in the cause of an illness. Many Western people are averse to these labels and the mere mention can trigger aggravation. Many don't want to hear what they have already heard from many other physicians, so if they don't mention conditions like stress or depression, I don't use them either. Instead, I try to bring about awareness without putting labels on their feelings. In contrast, Tibetan patients often accept their illnesses without much questioning. With them, I explain the cause of their medical condition so that they can come out of their illness. This, of course, is not meant to be a generalization, as each patient is treated individually, but is an example of how the physician's treatment differs from one culture to the other.

Also, to some patients, luck, karma, and merit are unfamiliar terms. In these cases, it's not helpful to bring up these ideas because it may be confusing and might lead them to lose confidence in the treatments. But when I have a patient who is familiar and comfortable with these concepts and presents with a disease that is not responding to the treatment, then I will discuss how the factors of karma, luck, and merit may be causing the illness. In such cases, the recovery is effective, faster, and has a positive impact on the patient's life.

When the disease becomes fatal, it is important not to reject the patient by saying things like, "There is nothing left to do." In these cases, I offer counseling and mentoring to help the patient bring about a change in mindset. This may help overcome the disease, as the healing power of the mind is most important. Each living moment is an opportunity to grow, to change our karma, and to increase merit, if not for this life, then for the next.

During my visit to Croatia in 2000, my tour organizers told me that I should avoid treating schizophrenic patients because of their mental volatility and the troubles that can result. I understood their concerns, but I told them that being a physician and healer meant it was my duty to assist every patient, and that I could counsel them with their diet, lifestyle, and emotional well-being. My intention is always to help all suffering patients equally. I don't know what the outcome will be in this life, but when there is an opportunity to help, it is important to follow through because in doing so, the luck, karma, and merits of the action may bring about a positive change in the patient's life.

Healing at the Time of Death

In the Tibetan tradition, the mental state at the time of dying is extremely important for the transition into the bardo. This is the reason why it is very important that physicians should help their patients die peacefully. A calm mind is very important when we die because we can have the opportunity to realize our own Buddha nature or transition to a fortunate birth in the next life. Traditional Tibetans believe in rebirth, and it is a very common practice to have Lamas or spiritual practitioners guide them towards a peaceful death.

My teacher, Dr. Trogawa Rinpoche, guided me in how to help dying patients. He taught me that the most important qualities for a physician at the time of death are unconditional love and compassion. You don't have to be an expert or a Lama; all you have to do is be naturally present with the patient—be there as a friend and offer comfort. This reassures patients and brings ease to their minds.

Rinpoche also taught me about the importance of focusing on the spiritual state with dying patients. He was not only a great physician and a monk but also a reincarnated Lama with great insight.

While I was training with Rinpoche, I encountered the following case: A healthy young woman went to visit her sister and when she found her sister wasn't home, she stopped at a neighbor's house for a drink of water. By the time she returned home, she wasn't feeling well. She quickly got worse and began to experience terrifying hallucinations. This frightened her mother, who then called me for help. At first, her mother thought that she was upset by something or was very tired. I was concerned her condition may well be something more serious, so I told Rinpoche about the case. He listened to the story, and then said that this problem was caused by the life force being stolen from her when she stopped at her sister's neighbors, and that her chance of survival was poor. He said it was more important to prepare her for a peaceful death than to try to cure the problem. Rinpoche advised doing three ritual practices in order to remove obstacles, strengthen her life force, and purify negative energies of the home and surrounding area. We also gave her medicine to calm her, as well as blessed medicine to remove negative energy and spirits. Being how very young and healthy she was, everyone was unprepared for her death, and so these rituals and treatments helped to calm the patient and her family. She did pass away, and she was quite peaceful at the time of death.

According to Tibetan Buddhist teachings, the state of mind at the time of death is extremely important. When the individual is calm and at peace, it helps them to not cling to this life. When someone is very scared or agitated, it can be very difficult to transition into the next life. We were able to help this young woman whose life was cut short so suddenly by helping her and her family to find ease and to accept death. It is very important to do everything we can to help patients and their families find some ease and peace during their transition to death.

Functions of the Physician's Mind

"The function of the Physician's mind is to engage in learning and the practice of healing without illusion, with full concentration, and with deep thought."

Being without illusion involves avoiding wrong views such as pride, jealousy, envy, aversion, or greed, and exhibiting the three aspects of intelligence—broad-mindedness, stable-mindedness, and deep-mindedness. Having all of these qualities combined with the experience of the medical theories, the mind will be free of confusion in the practice of medicine.

The physician must always maintain focus on their motivation for helping patients. In doing this, they will not become distracted from learning or practicing medicine. If our thinking becomes fearful or negative, it will inhibit treatment. Confidence plays a huge role in the effectiveness of healing. If the physician's mind is clear, positive, confident, and focused, the patient will gain confidence as well.

When referring to deep thinking, the physician does not think simply of temporarily relieving pains and aches, but of the holistic well-being of the patient. A person's experience of health depends on their physical, mental, emotional, social, and spiritual well-being. When treating a patient, it is beneficial to consider all of these.

THE SPECIFIC FUNCTIONS

"The three specific functions are view, meditation, and behavior."

The View

*"The Physician has a clear view of learning and
practicing the medical principles through the Middle
Path. This is done by avoiding the extreme thoughts
of neglectfulness, excessiveness, and adverseness.
Following the principle of a purely truthful mind in
the Middle Path is the best view of all."*

Avoiding extreme thoughts is the guiding principle in understanding and realizing the true nature of all phenomena
through the Middle Way. We do not view reality in terms of
right and wrong, or good and bad, but in terms of beneficial
and nonbeneficial depending on the situation. The physician
is not motivated to study and practice medicine in order to
become rich, famous, or powerful. The physician does not
care more for those who give extravagant gifts but treats all
with equanimity. Therefore, the physician maintains the goal
of benefiting others. In doing this, apathy, rigidity, and fanat-
icism are avoided. Being too strict in our beliefs creates problems with others who think differently. The physician accepts
all beings as their own loved ones, and tolerates various views,
as long as they are not harmful to others. When those views
do harm others, skillful means are used to encourage a change
in view.

In medical practice, maintaining the Middle Way is especially important while diagnosing and giving treatments.
Being neglectful, excessive, or adverse in diagnosis and treatment results in increasing the patient's suffering. For this reason, the physician practices the Middle Way. Neglectfulness
arises in the form of distractions and procrastinations that
impact the patient's diagnosis and treatment. Excessiveness
is when the physician spends too much time listening to

the patient's symptoms when the cause is clear, or when the physician gives excessive treatment to a disease that is mild in strength. Adverseness means holding wrong views about the patient, the disease, or the treatment. These include harboring feelings of sexual attraction or aversion towards the patient, being unconcerned for the patient's welfare, or misinterpreting the disease so that diagnosis and treatment will be ineffective.

The Middle Way also refers to the equanimity of the physician's mind. When someone offers praise, the physician doesn't get excited. If the patient says that the treatment is not working, the physician tries to adjust the treatment to better suit the disease without getting upset.

Upholding these views will prevent the wrongful treatment of the patient. This is why holding the Middle Path is considered to be supreme.

Meditation

"The meditative action is to practice the four limitless qualities of compassion, love, joy, and equanimity. And one does not practice the path of the four opposites."

The four limitless qualities of compassion, love, joy, and equanimity were explored in the section on the compassionate heart. Physicians are meant to continuously develop these qualities, as there is no limit to their depth.

The four opposites to these limitless qualities can simply be understood as direct antonyms. The opposite of limitless compassion is having no concern for others' welfare. The opposite of limitless love is wishing harm to others. The opposite of limitless joy is being angry or jealous of others' happiness. The opposite of limitless equanimity is attachment or aversion to others.

These four opposites can specifically be understood in the medical sense as well. There are different ways to interpret the four opposites. According to the Men-Tsee-Khang translation, the four opposites are: loving those who are ungrateful, being extra compassionate to those who hate religious doctrine and sentient beings, feeling joyful when a patient seen by another Physician dies, and not showing equanimity whether a patient survives or dies.

According to Trotrul Tsenam Rinpoche, the opposite of love is not caring about the suffering or death of a patient; the opposite of compassion is prioritizing financial gain when a patient takes a long time to heal; the opposite of joy is being happy when a patient dies, when a disease takes a long time to cure, or when there are many patients; and the opposite of equanimity is preferentially treating the rich, famous, or beautiful, and avoiding less pleasing patients.

The Behavior

> *"There are two categories of behaviors:*
> *Those which are to be avoided and those*
> *which are to be followed."*

Behavior to Be Avoided

> *"Refrain from the ten non-virtuous actions,*
> *as well as insanity, absurdity, conceit,*
> *sinfulness, and harmfulness."*

The ten non-virtuous actions are grouped into functions of the three gates: body, speech, and mind. The three non-virtuous actions of the body are killing, stealing, and sexual misconduct. Killing is intentionally taking the life of any living being. Stealing is taking the possessions of others without approval. Sexual misconduct is defined as any sexual behavior that can be harmful to oneself or others, such as having sexual relations with someone who does not consent, or with another's spouse, or with a patient.

The four non-virtuous functions of speech are lying, gossip, divisive speech, and harsh speech. Lying is telling falsehoods or obscuring the truth. Gossip is any type of meaningless talk. Divisive speech creates conflict, division, or discrimination among others, such as abusive speech based on race, ethnicity, gender, sexual identity, or religion. Harsh speech is speaking in ways that harm others, such as cursing another individual or society.

The three non-virtuous functions of the mind are envy, wishing harm to others, and holding a wrong view. Envy is wishing to have the good fortune, life, or possessions of others. Wishing harm to others includes imagining physical, mental, or emotional harm on another being. Holding a wrong view is not viewing the nature of reality as it truly is. Thinking of oneself as independent of others or thinking that material and phenomena are permanent, are both examples of wrong views. All of these actions are considered non-virtuous and will decrease merit.

Insanity in this context is not knowing the consequences of one's actions, and not knowing the difference between good and bad. An example of this would be a physician who behaves in a completely undisciplined manner, disregarding all social and cultural norms. This type of behavior should be avoided.

Absurdity is engaging in delusive and degenerative actions of body, speech, and mind. Here, physicians find enjoyment in meaningless activities and talk and don't follow through with commitments. They tend to exhibit laziness and spend too much time drinking alcohol or taking other drugs, which clouds both their awareness and conscience. Generally speaking, they don't work at benefiting others. These behaviors are to be avoided.

Conceit is thinking of ourselves as the greatest, and above all others. It also involves desiring material wealth beyond our means. Speaking badly of others, disgracing others, and not giving respect to others are also activities of conceit that the physician should avoid.

Sinfulness refers more to thoughtless actions and meaningless activities like giving treatment to a dead patient. It can also be considered sinful to claim spiritual powers that one does not have, or to casually swear in the name of God. It is basically doing something without a conscience.

Harmfulness is behaving in ways that harm others. It can be in the obvious sense of physical harm, by causing someone pain, suffering, or illness. It can also be done by thoughtless actions like borrowing other people's things and not taking care of them. Breaking the trust of our teachers, friends, relatives, and patients is also harmful behavior. Becoming too close or intimate with a patient can also be considered harmful behavior, because the attachment will interfere with the efficacy of the treatment. These types of behaviors should be avoided.

Behaviors to Be Followed

"The behaviors to be followed are the perfections
of generosity, morality, tolerance, and diligence in
healing to become a perfect Physician."

The behavior to be followed is based on the six perfections of Buddhist philosophy. The additional two perfections, meditative concentration and wisdom, are not mentioned but are assumed. There are four types of generosity, three types of morality, four types of patience, three types of diligence, three types of meditative concentration, and three types of wisdom. The following explanations come from the great sage, Desi Sangye Gyatso, in his *Blue Beryl* commentary on the *rGyud-bZhi*.

The Perfection of Generosity

The perfection of generosity is unconditional giving. Generosity of this sort comes in four types: material generosity, generosity of love, generosity that is without fear, and generosity of Dharma. Material generosity is simply the willingness to give others material things. For a physician, this form of generosity is in giving medicines and treatments without any conditions. This brings up the question of how giving medicines and treatments can be unconditional.

Traditionally, a physician did not request a specific fee for medical treatment. The treatment would be offered, and there was a cultural understanding that the patient would offer according to their own capacity as a gesture of gratitude. As mentioned above, it is taught to not treat patients who pay more with favoritism. The physician must try to keep the fees as moderate as possible in order to reach more patients across financial divides. If there are patients who truly show a great desire to get better and follow the physician's advice, but do not have the money to cover the cost of treatment, then the physician must try to help them.

The generosity of love is the caring, affectionate feeling that physicians hold for other sentient beings. Physicians can offer the same love and affection that they would give to their own child to their patients. Generosity without fear is the determination to bring others out of suffering no matter the personal sacrifices and consequences. In medical treatment, this means giving the correct treatment for any ailment without fear of the result. Generosity of Dharma is sharing the spiritual teachings and reading spiritual texts written by authentic masters. The generosity of Dharma is also about reciting healing mantras, reading the *rGyud-bZhi*, and sharing spiritual healing with others.

The Perfection of Morality

The perfection of morality involves three types of moral behavior—cultivating morality, morality of Dharma, and morality of others' well-being. In cultivating morality, the physician seeks to avoid the ten non-virtuous actions. Under the morality of Dharma, the physician adheres to the vows made to their teachers, maintains faith in the Three Jewels, and is disciplined in other meritorious actions such as the eightfold path. The morality of others' well-being is the discipline of working wholeheartedly for the benefit of others.

The Perfection of Tolerance

The perfection of tolerance is the ability to be patient in any situation. Tolerance has four types: tolerance of harmful beings, tolerance of Dharma, tolerance of suffering, and tolerance of the mind. The tolerance of harmful beings is the ability to withstand those that do harm to themselves and to others, without getting angry. The physician doesn't ignore the harm done by the action but avoids developing hate or anger towards the sentient being who committed the action. Tolerance in Dharma is the ability to be patient in the struggle of spiritual practice. Tolerance of suffering is the ability to bear our own suffering and the suffering of others. Tolerance of the mind is about being firm, confident, and fearless in the face of mental obscurations and situational difficulties.

The Perfection of Diligence

The perfection of diligence is when we find joy in working to benefit other sentient beings. There are three types of diligence: the diligence of accumulating merit, the diligence of responsibility, and the diligence of combining purposes. The diligence in accumulating merit is obtained by taking joy in activities that benefit both ourselves and others. The diligence of responsibility is when the physician undertakes the responsibility to relieve the suffering of others. The diligence of purpose is when the physician works continually for the benefit of their own self and all others without bias.

The Perfection of Meditative Concentration

The perfection of meditative concentration is being stable in mind, with complete focus, and with single-pointed concentration. There are three types of meditative concentration: the meditative concentration of residing in bliss, the meditative concentration of accomplishment, and the meditative concentration of performing with purpose.

Physicians are said to be in meditative concentration when they reside in the blissful and tranquil state of body and mind. The mind tends to create dualities of pleasure and pain, of health and disease, of rich and poor, of self and other, of samsara and nirvana. These dualities distract us from the truth of our Buddha nature, which is realized when we reach the perfection of meditative concentration and reside in great bliss. The physician is said to exhibit meditative concentration in the accomplishments of clairvoyance and other extraordinary spiritual attainments. And then, lastly, the physician is said to be in meditative concentration when performing with purpose and when working selflessly for the benefit of others.

The Perfection of Wisdom

The perfection of wisdom is to clearly understand the spiritual nature of all phenomena. This knowledge comes through the three aspects of wisdom: the wisdom of names, the wisdom of the name and meaning, and the wisdom attained through meditation. The practice of wisdom involves various stages depending on the practitioner's depth and intensity. Each stage is named based on the phenomena experienced.

The wisdom of names is to realize the appearance of phenomena, and to develop a complete understanding of how phenomena are labeled by the mind. These labels or names have the power to alter and influence our perception of the world and ourselves.

The wisdom of the name and meaning is to observe the name and appearance of phenomena while thinking of its true meaning. So here the label is observed and, at the same time, there is special attention paid to how that label is affecting the perception in the mind and senses.

The wisdom of meditation is to realize the true nature of phenomena without applying labels—to experience everything directly as it is.

Out of the six perfections, wisdom is the most important because it is inseparable from compassion on the path of enlightenment. With one of these alone, physicians cannot have full realization; they need both.

These perfections can be seen in the medical context as well. Physicians practicing wisdom and compassion are generous with their medicines, with treating patients, and with their medical advice. They maintain the morality of not engaging in practices that harm the patient and work solely for the benefit of the patient. This makes them tolerant in their practice, with their patient's suffering, and with their own personal suffering. Physicians are diligent in keeping updated with medical studies and medical practices, and continuously working for the benefit of patients. They practice meditative concentration while studying the medical history of patients, and while treating them, and do not become distracted or lazy. Finally, physicians exhibit wisdom in observing the nature of the patient's suffering and have clarity about how to treat them. These are the ways a physician practices the six perfections.

Recommendation for Practice: Gazing at Just One Object

Tibetan monks practice single-pointed meditation, which studies have found activates the frontal lobes of the brain. "These areas are associated with superior concentration and faster reaction time," says neuroscientist Dr. Brefczynski-Lewis. "The more a person meditates, the more they're able to concentrate on things with less effort."

Do It Yourself

You don't have to sit quietly for hours to reap brain gains, Brefczynski-Lewis says. Performing single-pointed meditation can be as easy as focusing on a single object as you're waiting in line at the supermarket!

"I have found that the greatest degree of inner tranquility comes from the development of love and compassion. The more we care for the happiness of others, the greater is our own sense of well-being. Cultivating a close, warmhearted feeling for others automatically puts the mind at ease. It is the ultimate source of success in life."
—His Holiness the Fourteenth Dalai Lama

Chapter 6

RESULTS OF THE PRACTICING PHYSICIAN

"There are two types of results of being a Physician—immediate and ultimate."

The results or fruits of a physician who is devoted to helping others out of suffering come within this life, and impact future lives as well. This is what is meant by immediate and ultimate.

THE IMMEDIATE RESULTS

"The immediate results provide happiness, power, prosperity, and joy in this life. Medical practice is the primary source to accomplish all these benefits, and so one shares the knowledge of healing with others. The Physician treats everyone equally and even treats harmful people as one's own relatives. The Physician examines the patient thoroughly with confidence and treats them accordingly, thereby earning merit and renown. The basic needs of the Physician are met without any struggle. At that time, the Physician should uphold the qualities of humility and modesty and accept the offerings. The

*Physician should accept whatever food and material
is offered when it is insisted upon, because later on
the gratitude may be forgotten."*

The immediate results of the medical practice all come within this life. Happiness is what each of us desires. This is a sense of satisfaction with our life and our work. Power is the spiritual accomplishment which results from right practice. Prosperity is the material comfort that is provided to the physician who works diligently and is generous. Joy is gained by seeing others being relieved of their suffering.

Medical practice which benefits the body and heals disease is the primary source for attaining these benefits. When physicians are able to accomplish this, they attain the fruits of happiness, satisfaction, prosperity, and joy. Realizing that this knowledge and practice will benefit others, the physician does not withhold the secrets of the medical practice. Instead, they share their knowledge with those who are willing to learn.

The physician does not only treat or teach those whom they like. They treat and teach anyone who is eager to learn, and anyone who is willing to help all sentient beings as though they are their own relatives. The physician examines medical students and patients thoroughly and offers teaching and guidance which they can understand, and which will benefit others as well. Any physician doing this achieves merit and an excellent reputation as a healer.

As mentioned earlier in this chapter, material wealth is not the goal of the physician. They always maintain humility and equanimity while practicing medicine. The food and material that is needed will come on its own, of this they can be sure. If they give up greediness, then the desires of the humble physician will easily be fulfilled. At the same time, if they accept the generosity and gratitude of others in the form of material, food, and money, it encourages the giver. If the physician doesn't accept the gratitude when it is being offered, it may be forgotten later.

THE ULTIMATE RESULTS

"The ultimate result of a Physician who has abandoned deceit and desires, and is totally focused on the practice of healing suffering beings, is the attainment of the highest state of Buddhahood. This is stated by Medicine Buddha, the King of Physicians."

The ultimate result is not just for this lifetime but goes beyond all concepts of life and death. It is stated by the Medicine Buddha that when the Physician has abandoned all negative actions, has completely tamed the mind to be free of the mental poisons, has infinitely developed the four limitless qualities, has actualized the six perfections, and is completely focused on healing others in their suffering, then the ultimate result is the highest state of Buddhahood. There is no better way to help suffering sentient beings than attaining this state!

Closing of the Physician Chapter

"After this discourse, the great sage, Rig-Pai-Yeshes, dissolved back into the crown chakra of the Medicine King. So ends the thirty-first chapter called 'Actions of a Physician' from 'The Explanatory Tantra' of the Nectar Essence of the Eight-Branch Secret Oral Instruction Tantra."

In the tradition of the *rGyud-bZhi*, the text describes the sage Rig-Pai-Yeshes dissolving back into the crown chakra because he is the manifestation of the wisdom of the Medicine Buddha. Some believe that the teachings are given by these sages to show how possible it is for each physician to attain the highest state of the Medicine Buddha, while others argue that this style of text shows that these are the direct teachings of the Buddha.

In another perspective, it is believed that the *rGyud-bZhi* was written by Yuthog Yonten Gonpo the Elder in the seventh century and later compiled and rewritten into its current form by Yuthog Yonten Gonpo the Younger in the eleventh century. This precious text remains unchanged today.

Recommendation for Practice: Laughing Out Loud

For thousands of years, many Tibetan monks have made a practice of laughing out loud after waking up, believing it makes them calmer and more focused. They are right. New studies have found that the act of laughter shuts off four different types of stress hormones, while also triggering the release of happiness-boosting endorphins. It also helps dilate capillaries in the head, which improves the flow of blood and oxygen to the brain.

Do It Yourself
Try laughing using different sounds and at different volumes: "ha-ha-ha," "hee-hee-hee," "ho-ho-ho," and so on. Studies show that simply faking a laugh gives you the same outcome and benefits as real laughter, since your body gets its physiological cues from the act of laughing itself.

"The planet does not need more successful people.
The planet desperately needs more peacemakers,
healers, restorers, storytellers,
and lovers of all kinds."
—His Holiness the Fourteenth Dalai Lama

CONCLUSION

"The Physician Chapter" teaches us how to be compassionate as physicians, healers, and healthcare practitioners. It teaches us how important the relationship between a physician and patient is. It also focuses on the transformation of ourselves through spiritual practice so that healing becomes perfected, culminating in freedom from the ignorance of samsara.

As emphasized earlier, the goal of Traditional Tibetan Medicine is to help our patients achieve a perfect state of balanced health by assessing their inner state and by detecting and healing imbalances or disorders within their physical, mental, emotional, and spiritual aspects, rather than just relieving their symptoms and pain. The physician works to restore the patient's health with the ultimate goal of bestowing true happiness and liberation from suffering.

However, if a physician's inner state is out of balance, can they effectively treat a patient? Therefore, physicians are strongly encouraged to maintain a healthy body, mind, and spirit in order to be ready and willing to help others. Making time for themselves, following a healthy diet and lifestyle, and doing spiritual practice will help the physician give patients the very best. Therefore, physicians must prepare their bodies and minds to become vessels of love and compassion. There is a Tibetan saying, "If one has a compassionate mind, everything (the earth and the path) will become compassionate as well."

Seeing patients only in terms of how much money can be earned will detract from the ability to help them and may result in a bad reputation and less money. Physicians who focus only on monetary profit and possess selfish motives at the heart of their practice will eventually encounter adverse consequences—this the law of cause and effect.

The rGyud-bZhi is taught to aspiring physicians who desire to heal the suffering of all sentient beings and to help them attain longevity and happiness through spiritual practices. This study will enable them to become respected physicians in society by their dedication, hard work, and holistic approach. In studying "The Physician Chapter" in depth, I hope you have enjoyed exploring the qualities, nature, definition, classification, functions, and results of the physician.

In the traditional manner of closing, I offer the following auspicious aspiration:

> *By this virtue*
> *May I quickly attain*
> *The highest state of Guru Medicine Buddha,*
> *And lead every single sentient being,*
> *Without exception, into the enlightened state!*

I wish and pray that all physicians, nurses, healthcare workers, healers, and readers learn and practice this profound teaching on "The Physician Chapter" in order to become compassionate beings and to attain complete Buddhahood.

GLOSSARY OF TERMS

Arura: The medicinal plant Terminalia chebula, often called the "King of Medicines" and held by the Medicine Buddha.

Ayurveda: An Indian system of medicine that means "the science of healing" in Sanskrit.

Baidur sNgon-Po (Blue Beryl): A commentary on the *rGyud-bZhi* written by Desi Sangye Gyatso in the seventeenth century.

Badkan: Phlegm, the combination of earth and water elements in the body.

Bardo: "An in-between state." Most commonly refers to the state between death and rebirth. There are four Bardos: life, dying, death, and becoming.

Bodhichitta: Sanskrit term for "the mind of enlightenment." In Tibetan, it is called *Jangchup Sempa*; in English, "Buddha mind."

Bon: The civilization of Tibet that existed prior to the introduction of Buddhism.

Buddha: An awakened and realized being. Also refers to Shakyamuni, the founder of Buddhism.

Chagpori: Refers to the mountain where the first official medical college in Tibet was located. The full name of the medical college was "Chagpori Dro Phen Ling Dratsang" (the Iron Mountain Monastery for Benefiting Sentient Beings).

Chog-She: Contentedness.

Dam-Tshig: Pure Intention.

Desi Sangye Gyatso: The regent to the great Fifth Dalai Lama who was a renowned scholar of Tibetan Medicine and Astrology. His texts and commission of the original seventy-nine medical thankas have been pivotal to the study of Tibetan Medicine.

Dhamchen Degu: The nine protector deities of Tibetan Medicine.

Dharma: A spiritual path involving spiritual teachings, or the teachings of Buddha.

Dung gi Thor Chog: "Crowned with a Conch." Name of the first physician in the royal lineage of Tibetan physicians.

Eight Branches of Traditional Tibetan Medicine: Body, Pediatric, Gynecology, Evil spirit, Wounds, Toxicology, Geriatrics, and Infertility.

Eight Medicine Buddhas: Excellent Name, Precious One, Stainless Excellent Gold, Supreme Glory Free From Sorrows, Melody Ocean of Dharma, King of Clear Knowing, Medicine Buddha, and Buddha Shakyamuni.

Eightfold Path: Right View, Right Resolve, Right Speech, Right Conduct, Right Livelihood, Right Effort, Right Mindfulness, and Right Meditation.

Eighteen Fields of Knowledge: Music, lovemaking, sustenance, arithmetic, grammar, medicine, behavior, fine arts, archery, logic, yoga, study, recollection, astronomy, astrology, optical aberrations, antiquity, and history.

Eighty Minor Signs of a Buddha: Nails are copper-colored; nails are moderately shiny; nails are raised; nails are round; nails are broad; nails are tapered; veins do not protrude; veins are free of knots; ankles do not protrude; feet are not uneven; walks with a lion's gait; walks with an elephant's gait; walks with the gait of a goose; walks with a bull's gait; gait tends to the right; gait is elegant; gait is steady; body is well-covered; body looks as if it were polished; body is well-proportioned;

body is clean and pure; body is smooth; body is perfect; body contains the full set of thirty-two signs of an enlightened body; physical bearing is excellent and dignified; steps are even; eyes are perfect; is youthful; body is not sunken; body is broad; body is not loose; limbs are well-proportioned; vision is clear and not blurred; belly is round; belly is perfectly moderate; belly is not long; belly does not bulge; navel is deep; navel winds to the right; perfectly handsome; habits are clean; body is free of moles and discoloration; hands are soft as cotton wool; lines on palms are clear; lines on palms are deep; lines on palm are long; face is not too long; lips are red like copper; tongue is pliant; tongue is thin; tongue is red; voice is like thunder; voice is sweet and gentle; teeth are round; teeth are sharp; teeth are white; teeth are even; teeth are tapered; nose is prominent; nose is clean; eyes are clear and wide; eyelashes are thick; black and white parts of eyes are well-defined and like lotus petals; eyebrows are long; eyebrows are smooth; eyebrows are soft; eyebrows are evenly haired; hands are long and extended; ears are of equal size; ear sense power is perfect; forehead is well-formed and well-defined; forehead is broad; head is very large; hair is black as a bumblebee; hair is thick; hair is soft; hair is untangled; hair is not unruly; hair is fragrant; hands and feet are marked with auspicious emblems such as the srivasta and svastika.

Eleven Sections of Learning: Summary, Formation of Body, Pathology, Behavioral Regimens, Dietary Regimens, Pharmacology, Medical Instruments, Maintenance of Health, Diagnostic Approaches, Method of Healing, and Practicing Physician.

Fifteen Occasions of Healing: Healing the Three Humors, Healing Internal Disorders, Healing Hot Disorders, Healing the Upper Body, Healing Vital and Vessel Organ Disorders, Healing Genital Disorders, Healing Unclassified Disorders,

Healing Disorders which Simultaneously Develop Lesions, Healing Pediatric Disorders, Healing Gynecological Disorders, Healing Evil Spirits Disorders, Healing Wounds, Healing Toxicities, Healing Geriatrics Disorders, and Healing Infertility.

Five Biles: Digestive, color-transforming, accomplishing, visual, and complexion-clearing.

Five Phlegms: Supporting, decomposing, experiencing, satisfying, and connecting.

Five Winds: Life-sustaining, ascending, pervasive, fire-accompanying, and descending.

Four Limitless Qualities: Compassion, love, joy, and equanimity.

Four Opposites: Compassion to the ungrateful people, loving those who hate religious doctrines, being joyful towards others' mistakes, and being biased towards partiality.

Four Sutras of Explanation: Pulse and Urine Examination, Pacifying Medications, Evacuative Therapies, and Mild and Drastic External Therapies.

Four Tantras (of *rGyud-bZhi*): "The Root Tantra," "The Explanatory Tantra," "The Secret Tantra," and "The Last Tantra."

Four Types of Generosity: Material, love, fearlessness, and Dharma.

Four Types of Tolerance: Tolerance of harmful beings, tolerance of Dharma, tolerance of suffering, and tolerance of the mind.

gDon: Spirits.

Jivaka Kumara: Referred to as the first physician of the Buddhist lineage, and physician disciple of the historical Buddha.

Kalachakra: Highest spiritual empowerment of Vajrayana Buddhism that is meant for world peace and harmony.

Karma: "Action." The law of cause and effect. In Tibetan, it is called "Las" (pronounced *Ley*).

Khenrab Norbu: A great scholar of Tibetan Medicine, the first director of the Lhasa Men-Tsee-Khang, and personal physician to the Thirteenth Dalai Lama.

King Trisong Detsen: The thirty-eighth king of Tibet, renowned as one of the three "Dharma Kings of Tibet" and for inviting the Buddhist master, Padmasambhava, from India to Tibet. He was responsible for the building of the Samye Monastery. During his rule, he organized one of the first international medical conferences in Tibet.

Lama: "No one above." An honorific title used for a monk, nun, or spiritual teacher.

Lha-rJe: "God King," a term of respect given to physicians.

Loong (Lung): Spiritual transmission.

Lopon Shanglon: One of the nine protector deities of Tibetan Medicine, who is often depicted in the center of images of the protectors.

Marigpa: Ignorance, or without wisdom.

Men-Pa (sMan-Pa): "A physician." One who heals the body, speech, and mind.

Menrampa: "Eminent physician." After ten years of practice Tibetan physicians become eligible for the Menrampa degree by receiving additional medical training and passing the examination.

Men-Tsee-Khang: The Tibetan Medical and Astrological Institute. There are two Men-Tsee-Khang: one, located in Lhasa, Tibet, was founded by the Thirteenth Dalai Lama in 1916; the other, in Dharamsala, India, was founded by His Holiness the Fourteenth Dalai Lama in 1961.

Middle Path: The spiritual path set forth by the historical Buddha, which is without extremes.

mKhris-pa: Bile, fire element or heat in the body.

Naga: "Serpent water spirit" in Sanskrit, *gLu* in Tibetan.

Nagarjuna: A great scholar of Buddhism and medicine.

Nine Protector Deities: Nyod Jin Chen Po Dud Dul, Eka Zita Ma, Sog Gi Pu Dri, Khyab Jug Chen Po, Dadrul Jig Jed, Che Jang Chu Mar, Shanti Nag Po, Shan Pa Mar Nag, and Hab Se Las Khen.

Nirvana: Liberation or enlightenment.

Ngon-Shes: Clairvoyance.

Nod-ja: "That which is harmed," referring to the bodily constituents and the excretions.

Nod-jed: "That which harms," referring to the three humors: rLung, mKhris-pa and Badkan.

Reincarnated Lama: The reincarnation of high Lamas or spiritual teachers has been recognized within the Tibetan Buddhist tradition for a very long time. These masters develop the mind of enlightenment so strongly that it is carried into the next birth. These masters can then continue in the selfless work of a bodhisattva, for the sake of sentient beings. They are recognized by their actions, characteristics, and even memories from a previous life. On some occasions, these powerful masters can predict when and where they will be reborn. On other occasions, specific divinations are performed so that the new incarnation of a previous teacher can be found.

rGyud-bZhi: "The four tantras or treatises." It is the short name for the fundamental medical text of Traditional Tibetan Medicine, which has the full title of *Dutsi Nyingpo Yenlag Gyepa Sangwa Manga Gyi Gyud* (Nectar Essence of the Eight Branch Secret Oral Instruction Tantra).

Rig-pai-Yeshes: A sage manifested from the Medicine Buddha whose name means "Light of Wisdom"

Rinpoche: "Precious One." An honorific title used for a highly respected spiritual master.

rLung: Wind, the air element, which moves through the body.

rLung-rTa: "Wind horse." An ancient shamanic term that refers to luck or fortune.

Samsara: The cycle of birth and death.

Sampa Karwa: "White mind" or "compassionate heart." It refers to the love, compassion, joy, and equanimity that make up the mind of enlightenment.

Sangha: The Dharma friends and followers of the teachings of Buddha.

Sangye Menla: "The Medicine Buddha." Also "Unsurpassed Perfect Healer" and "King of Physicians."

Six Perfections: Generosity, morality, tolerance, diligence, meditative concentration, and wisdom.

Six Realms: God, demi-god, human being, hell, hungry ghost, and animal.

Six Types of Clairvoyance: Divine seeing, divine hearing, knowledge of others' thoughts and emotions, knowledge of miracles, knowledge of past and future, and knowledge of decay and destruction.

Sowa Rigpa: "The science of healing," the Traditional Tibetan Medical system.

Stupa: A form or monument that represents the mind of the Buddha, which is blessed and filled with consecrated ingredients and prayers.

Tantra: A treatise or text containing spiritual and healing instructions.

Ten Directions of the Universe: East, West, North, South, North-East, North-West, South-East, South-West, Up, and Down.

Ten Non-virtuous Actions: Three of the body—killing, stealing, and sexual misconduct; four of speech—lying, gossiping, divisive speech, and harsh speech; three of the mind—envy, wishing harm of others, and holding a wrong view.

Terton: "Treasure revealer." One who reveals spiritual texts and teachings.

Thangka: Tibetan spiritual paintings depicting deities, Buddhas, bodhisattvas, and sages. Seventy-nine medical thangkas were commissioned by Desi Sangye Gyataso in the seventeenth century, and have become invaluable teaching tools for students and scholars of Tibetan medicine.

Thirty-Two Major Signs of Buddha: Palms of hands and feet bear signs of a wheel; feet are well-set upon the ground like a tortoise; fingers and toes are webbed; palms of hands and soles of feet are smooth and tender; body has seven prominent features: broad heels, broad hands, broad shoulder blades, and broad neck; fingers are long; heels are soft; body is tall and straight; ankle bones do not protrude; hairs on body point upward; ankles are like an antelope's; hands are long and beautiful; private organ is withdrawn; body is the color of gold; skin's thin and smooth; each hair curls to the right; face is adorned by a coiled hair between eyebrows; upper part of body is like that of a lion; head and shoulders are perfectly round; shoulders are broad; has an excellent sense of taste, even of the worst tastes; body has the proportions of a banyan tree; has a protrusion on the crown of head; tongue is long and thin; voice is mellifluous; cheeks are like those of a lion; teeth are white; no gaps between teeth; teeth are evenly set; has a total of 40 teeth; eyes are the color of a sapphire; eyelashes are like those of a magnificent heifer.

Three Gates: The body, speech, and mind.

Three Jewels: Buddha, Dharma and Sangha.

Three Types of Diligence: The diligence of accumulating merit, the diligence of responsibility, and the diligence of combining purposes.

Three Types of Firm-Mindedness: The firm-mindedness

of residing in bliss, the firm-mindedness of accomplishment, and the firm-mindedness of performing with purpose.

Three Types of Intelligence: Broad-mindedness, stable-mindedness, and deep-mindedness.

Three Methods of Diagnosis: Seeing, feeling, and questioning.

Three Types of Morality: Cultivating morality, morality of Dharma, and morality of others' well-being.

Three Poisons: Desire, aversion, and delusion.

Three Stages of a Compassionate Heart: Preliminary practice, main practice, and dedication practice.

Three Types of Wisdom: The wisdom of names, the wisdom of the name and meaning, and the wisdom attained through meditation.

Tonglen (gTong Len): The Buddhist practice of exchanging one's own happiness for the suffering of others through meditation as guided by a spiritual master.

Tri ('Khrid): Spiritual explanation.

Tsug Lha Khang: His Holiness the Fourteenth Dalai Lama's main temple in Dharamsala, India.

Twelve Defects of the Inferior Physician: A physician without lineage, a physician who does not know the meaning of the text, a physician without experience, a physician who does not know the diagnostic methods, a physician who does not know the pulse and urine analysis, a physician who cannot speak confidently, a physician who does not know the treatment methods, a physician who does not know dietary and lifestyle behaviors, a physician who does not know the administration of pacifying compounds, a physician who does not know the action of cleansing therapies, a physician who does without medicines and medical instruments, and a physician who does not know venesection and cauterization techniques.

Two-Fold Recognition: Mahayana and Hinayana.

Two Sages: Rig-pai-Yeshes (Wisdom Light), originally was said to emanate from the Buddha's heart in "The Root Tantra," but later in "The Explanatory Tantra," was said to emanate from Buddha's crown. Yid-les-sKyes (Born of the Mind), was said to emanate from the Medicine Buddha's tongue.

Vajra: The symbol of combining wisdom and compassion that is often translated as "diamond" or "lightning."

Vajrayana: "The diamond path." A form of Mahayana Buddhism predominant in Tibet.

Wang (dBang): Spiritual empowerment.

Yid-les-s Kyes: A sage manifested from the Medicine Buddha whose name means "Born of the Mind."

Yoga: A traditional practice of uniting the body and mind to bring about a perfect state of health.

Yuthog Nying-Thig Nyam-Len: The spiritual practice of Tibetan physicians, which was taught by Yuthog Yonten Gonpo, the Younger.

Yuthog Yonten Gonpo, the Elder: Commonly called the "Father of Tibetan Medicine," he was a great master and the author of the *rGyud-bZhi*.

Yuthog Yonten Gonpo, the Younger: Great physician, scholar, and spiritual teacher of Tibetan Medicine who lived during the eleventh century. He compiled and rewrote the present form of the *rGyud-bZhi* and taught the Yuthog Nying-Thig spiritual practice.

BIBLIOGRAPHY

Primary Sources

Gyatso, Desi Sangye. *gSo-ba Rig-pa' bsTan-bCho sMan-bLa' dGongs-rGyen rGyud-bZhi' gSal-Byed Baidur sNgon-Poi'Malli-ka.* 2008. Dharamsala, India: Men-Tsee-Khang Translation Department.

Yonten Gompo, Yuthog, *The Basic and The Explanatory Tantra for the Quintessential Instructions on the Eight Branches of the Ambrosia Tantra.* 2008. Dharamsala, India: Men-Tsee-Khang Translation Department.

Yonten Gonpo, Yuthog. *bDud-rTsi sNying-po Yan-Lag brGyad-pa gSang-ba Man-Ngag Gi rGyud.* 1980. Lhasa, Tibet. Bod-lJongs Mi-dMangs dPe-sKrun Publishing Company.

Tsenam Rinpoche, Troru. *gSo-rig rGyud-bZhi 'Grel-Chen Drang-Srong Shel-Lung.* 2000. Lhasa: Si-Khron Mi-Rig dPe-sKrun.

Secondary Sources

Beer, Robert. *The Handbook of Tibetan Buddhist Symbols.* 2003. Chicago: Serindia Publications, Inc.

Chokyi Nyima Rinpoche, and Shlim, David R. *Medicine and Compassion.* 2004. Somerville, MA: Wisdom Publications, Inc.

Clark, Barry. *The Quintessence Tantras of Tibetan Medicine.* 1995. Ithaca, NY: Snow Lion Publications.

Dalai Lama, His Holiness, and Howard C. Cutler. *The Art of Happiness.* 1998. New York: Riverhead Books.

Dalai Lama, His Holiness, and Jefferey Hopkins. *How to Be Compassionate.* 2007. London: Rider Books.

Dalai Lama, His Holiness. *Power of Compassion.* 1995. London: Thorsons Publications.

Das, Sarat Chandra. *A Tibetan-English Dictionary.* 1902. Calcutta, India: The Bengal Secretariat Book Depot.

Doidge, Norman. *The Brain That Changes Itself.* 2007. New York: Viking Penguin.

Dondhen, Yeshi. *Health Through Balance: An Introduction to Tibetan Medicine.* 1986. Ithaca, NY: Snow Lion Publications.

Dorjee, Dr. Pema, Jones, Janet and Moore, Terrence. *The Spiritual Medicine of Tibet: Heal Your Spirit, Heal Yourself.* 2005. London: Watkins Books.

Emoto, Masaru. *The Hidden Messages of Water,* 2004. New York: Atria Books.

Hustedt Crook, Barbara. "Tibetan Joy Secrets: Less Stress, More Happiness." *Woman's World Magazine.* February 9, 2009. pp. 40-41.

Ricard, Matthieu, *Happiness: A Guide to Developing Life's Most Important Skill.* 2007. London: Atlantic Books.

Ricard, Matthieu. *Altruism.* 2015. London: Atlantic Books.

Swanson, Eric, Rinpoche, Yongey Mingyur. *The Joy of Living.* 2007. New York: Random House, Inc.

Tsona, Dr. Lobsang Tsultrim, Dakpa, Dr. Tenzin. *Fundamentals of Tibetan Medicine.* 2001. Dharamsala, India: Men-Tsee-Khang Editorial & Publication Dept.

Sarva Mangalam
(*May All Be Well*)

ACKNOWLEDGMENTS

I am very grateful to the late Dr. Trogawa Rinpoche, who was the founder and director of Chagpori Tibetan Medical Institute in Darjeeling, India, for his generosity in giving me special admission to study Traditional Tibetan Medicine. I am also thankful to Dr. Tenzin Dakpa Rishing, both for being my teacher at Chagpori and for suggesting that I join the institute.

The late Dr. Walburg Maric Oeheler, president of the German Acupuncture Society, sponsored my medical studies at Chagpori, and the late Dr. Lobsang Chophel taught me as a private student at Men-Tsee-Khang in Dharamsala, India.

My deep gratitude to Mr. Tempa Tsering, former minister for the Central Tibetan Administration and director of India and East Asia Office of His Holiness the Dalai Lama, who inaugurated my center, the Tibetan Healing and Wellness Center, in Bangalore, India, and gave me invaluable support and guidance.

This book would not have been possible without my student, Kyle Weaner (Tenzin Samdup), whose hard work and dedication toward learning Traditional Tibetan Medicine inspired me to write this book. His mother, Barbara Weaner, has also been a source of constant encouragement for me. I am also deeply grateful to Charlene D. Jones, a psychotherapist and longtime Buddhist practitioner, for supporting my family since the passing of my father when I was twelve years old. I'm equally thankful for her suggestions for the book, including her inspiring me to correlate neuroscience with Traditional Tibetan Medicine so that this work may benefit larger audiences. And I am very grateful to the neuroscientist Dr. Julie Brefczynski-Lewis, my Dharma friend and colleague, for her contributions here relating to the field of neuroscience.

I sincerely thank the late Dr. Pema Dorjee, senior physician of Traditional Tibetan Medicine and author of the book *The Spiritual Medicine of Tibet: Heal Your Spirit, Heal Yourself*, for giving me the opportunity to do my internship under his guidance in 1998, and for graciously giving feedback on my manuscript. Thanks also to the late Dr. Satish Inamdar, who was an oncologist, director of Krishnamurthy Foundation in Bangalore, India, and author of the book *Mahatma Gandhi and His Holiness the Dalai Lama On Non-Violence and Compassion*, for offering his valuable suggestions on my manuscript.

I extend my heartfelt thanks to Dr. Tsewang Tamdin (visiting physician to His Holiness the Fourteenth Dalai Lama), Geshe Dorji Damdul (director of Tibet House, New Delhi), Matthieu Ricard (Buddhist monk, scientist, translator, and author), Dr. Dorjee Rapten Neshar (chief medical officer of Men-Tsee-Khang, Bangalore), and Dr. Sonam Dorjee (Science Pala) for reading my manuscript and for their feedback.

Thanks to the former editor of Snow Lion Publications, Sidney Piburn, for his confidence and guidance, as well as Annie Bien, Jacob David, Kelly Alba, and Lisbeth Miller for assistance in editing the manuscript. Thanks to Terri Nash, Ellen Scordato, Nirmala Govindarajan, and Jasmine Shah for their unfailing support. A special thanks to Lisbeth and Tod Miller for their generosity, guidance, and support.

I express my gratitude to my loving mother, the late Tsering Norzom, for her faith in me and her patience in allowing me to study for as long as I wanted. And finally, my heartfelt thanks to my wife, Rinzing Dolma, and my two sons, Tenzin Yonten and Tenzin Rigzin Yonten, for being my strength and inspiration to complete this book. And last but not least, I thank all my well-wishers for their support and prayers.

—*Dr. Jampa Yonten*

ABOUT THE AUTHOR

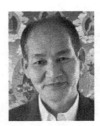 Dr. Jampa Yonten has been very fortunate to receive the Medicine Buddha initiation three times from His Holiness the Fourteenth Dalai Lama: once during the Kalachakra initiation at Jispa in Himachal Pradesh in 1994, then at Sera Monastery, Bylakuppe, in 2009, and finally in Dharamsala at the Tsug Lha Khang (Main Temple), organized by the Central Council of Tibetan Medicine, in 2014. He has also received the Medicine Buddha initiation from His Eminence Khamtrul Rinpoche while working in Dharamsala, and from his teacher, Dr. Trogawa Rinpoche, who also bestowed the transmission, empowerment, and explanation of the Yuthog Nyingthig. In 2009, Dr. Yonten again received the Yuthog Nyingthig transmission and empowerment from His Eminence Taglung Tsetrul Rinpoche, which also was organized by the Central Council of Tibetan Medicine in Dharamsala.

Dr. Yonten graduated from Chagpori Tibetan Medical Institute, in Darjeeling, and had the privilege of working under senior eminent Tibetan physicians such as Dr. Trogawa Rinpoche, Dr. Pema Dorjee, Dr. Thubten Gyatso (Tholing Rinpoche), Dr. Yeshi Dorjee, and Dr. Kyizom (Mundgod). Dr. Yonten successfully completed the Menrampa degree from Men-Tsee-Khang in 2010. He currently heads the

Tibetan Healing and Wellness Center in Bangalore, India, and travels around the world for consultations, teachings, and healing retreats.

ABOUT THE COAUTHOR

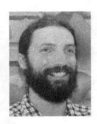 Kyle Weaner (Tenzin Samdrup) is a student of Dr. Jampa Yonten and a Tibetan medical practitioner, massage therapist, and yoga teacher. He studied Traditional Tibetan Medicine under Dr. Yonten as an apprentice from 2004 to 2012 and received the Medicine Buddha initiation from His Holiness the Fourteenth Dalai Lama in 2009 at Sera Monastery in Bylakuppe, India, and from His Holiness the Seventeenth Karmapa in 2008 at Karma Thegsum Chöling monastery in Shamong Township, New Jersey. He is the founder and director of the Jivaka Wellness Center in Elkins, West Virginia.

CPSIA information can be obtained
at www.ICGtesting.com
Printed in the USA
JSHW081416210323
39181JS00001B/1